Aromatherapy and the Mind

By the same author

The Encyclopaedia of Essential Oils
Home Aromatherapy
Lavender Oil
Rose Oil
Tea Tree Oil

AROMATHERAPY AND THE MIND

Thorsons
An Imprint of HarperCollins*Publishers*

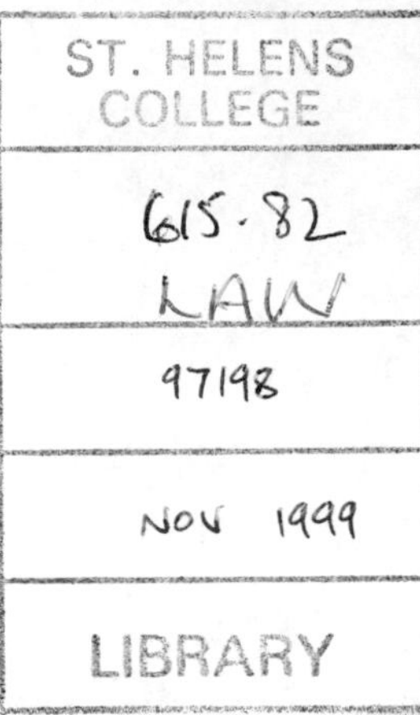

Thorsons
An Imprint of HarperCollins*Publishers*
77–85 Fulham Palace Road,
Hammersmith, London W6 8JB

First published by Thorsons 1994
This edition 1998
10 9 8 7 6 5

A catalogue record for this book
is available from the British Library

ISBN 0 7225 2927 9

Printed and bound in Great Britain by
Woolnough Bookbinding Limited, Irthlingborough, Northamptonshire

TO ALEC

Contents

FOREWORD

Aromatherapy and the Mind explores the impact of scent on human consciousness throughout history. Part I asserts that scent is not only therapeutic and aesthetic, but profoundly psychoactive. It examines the way that botanical aromatics evolved through the use of incense, perfume, the symbolic imagination and psycho-aromatherapy. We are introduced to ancient fragrant myths, magic and romance, as well as modern aromatic psychology and science.

This book is an aromatic treasure chest, for there is a wealth of information here. It is peppered with apt literary quotations and redolent poetic images. Part II is a compilation of the psychoactive and therapeutic properties of specific oils and an excellent complement to Lawless's earlier work, *The Encyclopaedia of Essential Oils*. For those interested in the history of aromatic psychology, *Aromatherapy and the Mind* presents a captivating cross-cultural overview beginning with Sumeria, Egypt, Greece and Rome. A central theme of the book is concerned with archaic magical-alchemical consciousness and how it was supplanted by scientific materialism, culminating in the mind/body split of the seventeenth-century scientific revolution.

Within the last 20 years we have seen the emergence of a new paradigm which has been reflected in literature and lecture theaters by a new physics, a new biology, a new botany, a new archaeology and a new aromatics. What makes each of these disciplines 'new' is the addition of mind and conscious awareness to their knowledge base. Not 'mind' in a limited sense as the mental power of logical thought, but 'mind' in a more expanded sense which includes spirit. Mind in this larger view animates and interacts with the physical environment, which it can either make sacred or desecrate. This knowledge is ancient and is evident in magic, meditation and early forms of religion.

Paradoxically, this new dimension of mind is also what reconnects each of these contemporary disciplines to their ancient roots before there was a division between psyche and soma. Today there is an intuition within the aromatherapy community to remember the severed links between mind, body and fragrance. This trend is part of the olfactory renaissance. *Aromatherapy and the Mind* puts this renaissance in historical perspective.

I met Julia when English aromatherapy was still in its infancy. We share an aromatic lineage. Her mother Kerttu Smith, a Finnish biochemist, introduced me to the fragrant virtues of aromatic oils which I distributed for her company Natural Essence in London.

In 1982 when I met Kerttu, I was a visiting lecturer in megalithic archaeology and general systems theory at the School of Environmental Studies, University of London. Among the libraries that I frequented was the Warburg Institute. This unique collection specializes in texts and studies of the survival of classical antiquity in the civilization of Western Europe. The library was a delight to explore. It exuded an almost monastic ambience of hushed silence and academic reflection. Thus when Julia told me that she had done her historical aromatic research at the Warburg Institute, I could relate to the seasoned atmosphere in which this book took root and blossomed.

Aromatherapy and the Mind is a scholarly bouquet for us, an impressive distillation of aromatic history and psychology. It will be especially rewarding for those practitioners who have absorbed and already practice 'the lavender-for-headaches' level of aromatherapy and desire more knowledge about the subtle effects of aromatherapy on the mind.

John J. Steele
Lifetree Aromatix
Sherman Oaks, California
November, 1993

Acknowledgements

Aromatherapy and the Mind has not been an easy book to write ... like the nature of the mind itself, perfume has a subtle and elusive quality. I am aware that the information presented here simply represents the tip of an iceberg. The vast majority of questions regarding the psychological effects of fragrance remain unanswered, for in the interaction between mind and scent, personal and transpersonal elements are both brought into play. As Maurice Rogers, the President of Dior Perfumes, has observed:

> Scent, even in hard, materialistic times like these, still offers a direct route to the unconscious ... perfume is one of the last territories of the irrational. The deep aim of perfumery is to find ingredients that will open new doors.

Likewise, rather than providing conclusive answers, this book consequently takes the form of an exploration, an invitation to 'open new doors'. It is also my hope that in the future, natural aromatics will be used increasingly for their psychological benefits, as essential oils come to be recognized for their multi-faceted healing potential.

I would especially like to thank all the following people who have helped or contributed to this project in a variety of ways:

Noel Cobb, Carola Beresford-Cooke, John Black, Tristram Hull, Nicole Perez, Jill Purce, Claire and John Sharkey and Rupert Sheldrake for sending me relevant articles and information; Angelica Bradley and Dorothea Vincentz for translating chunks of material from foreign texts; Judy Allan, Jane Graham-Maw and those at Thorsons for their writing and editorial advice; Cara Denman for her guidance; John Steele for reading the text through at manuscript stage, for his astute comments and for writing the Foreword; Robert Bly for his kind permission to reprint 'The Wind One Brilliant Day...'; and, last but not least, my friends and family who have given their support – Ute and Myles Lawless, Sue Mitchell, Len Smith, my husband Alec and daughter Natasha.

Introduction

> And so he would now study perfumes ... He saw that there was no mood of the mind that had not its counterpart in the sensuous life, and set himself to discover their true relations, wondering what there was in frankincense that made one mystical, and in ambergrise that stirred one's passions, and in violets that woke the memory of dead romances, and in musk that troubled the brain, and in champak that stained the imagination; and seeking often to elaborate a real psychology of perfumes, and to estimate the several influences of sweet smelling roots, and scented pollen-laden flowers, or aromatic balms, and of dark and fragrant woods, of spikenard that sickens, of hovenia that makes men mad, and of aloes that are said to be able to expel melancholy from the soul.
>
> Oscar Wilde, *The Picture of Dorian Gray*, 1891

Aromatherapy and the Mind is an exploration into the realm of fragrance. Throughout the history of civilization, perfumes, incense, aromatic plants and oils have been used to enhance human experience in many different cultures, both ancient and modern. For although the term 'aromatherapy' is new, the practice of using aromatics not only as physical remedies but also to influence the mind and the emotions is an ancient art. From the earliest times, herbs have been used as magic amulets, to protect from evil spirits or to bring good fortune; incense has traditionally been burnt at religious or ritual occasions to help transport the mind to another dimension; perfumes have been created to enrapture prospective lovers with their fragrance; and the power of essential oils has long been associated with alchemy and the quest for an 'elixir of life'.

The revival of interest in aromatics and the modern day enthusiasm for aromatherapy are, I believe, due to a combination of factors. Firstly, like many other 'alternative' treatments, aromatherapy represents a return to nature, and embraces an environmental awareness and a holistic approach. Secondly, the oils are pleasant and easy to use, they are highly concentrated and require little or no preparation, thereby fitting in with the fast pace of modern life. Lastly, aromatics are not simply physical remedies – they also affect the emotions and deeper levels of the human psyche, a factor which many people sense intuitively. Due to their psycho-active properties, essential oils can help to combat the emotional instability and inner disillusionment which lie at the root of so much of the dis-ease manifest in contemporary life.

Since the malaise of our present day culture in the West is largely based on fundamental social and environmental problems, such as the breakdown of the nuclear family, the long-term effects of materialism, the decline of spiritual or moral values and the destruction of the ecosystem, individuals are now searching for new ways of dealing with this crisis – ways that do not contribute further to the existing problems. Stress, in the form of depression, anxiety or hyperactivity, is one of the most common problems encountered today, and it is an area in which aromatherapy enjoys a great deal of success, especially when it is combined with massage. This is because it works on a variety of different levels, including the non-rational. Scent can help us to reconnect with our emotional interior and to transform it. More and more people are becoming intrigued by the psychological potential of fragrance, not least because of the immediacy of its effect. The direct way in which a scent can bring back memories from years ago, quite suddenly and as clear as daylight, is a common occurrence, yet quite inexplicable. Everyone has had such experiences, pleasing or otherwise. I myself cannot smell pine resin without remembering my early childhood in Finland, and the aroma of the pine logs and timber in the sauna.

In *Aromatherapy and the Mind* the reader is invited to explore their own relationship with the sensation of smell. We each acquire a vast vocabulary of odours, yet to a large degree we remain unconscious of how we are conditioned by our response to particular scents. It could even be said that there has developed something of a taboo about our reaction to certain aromas, especially with regard to the sexual messages they convey. The recent novel *Perfume: The Story of a Murderer* by Patrick Süskind is a macabre insight into the vision of a man obsessed by his remarkable sense of smell and intoxicated by its power.

But how much is an individual influenced by fragrance, how does it work and can it be used effectively to bring about predictable results? Much of the current research which is being carried out into the effects of aromatic oils and the role of fragrance indicates that it is a very powerful tool indeed! Rovesti describes the response of psychiatric patients to aromatherapy:

> It may be said that the patients feel as if transported by the perfume or by the essential oil into a different, more agreeable and acceptable world, so that many of their reactive instincts are curbed and they gradually return towards normality.

Current research into the effects of certain essential oils on brainwave patterns and their ability to sedate or stimulate the nervous system as a whole has also brought forth some interesting results. If these effects can be proven, aromatherapy may provide a valuable alternative to some types of orthodox drug treatment. According to the psychologist William Cain of Yale, the twenty-first century will be the era of scent:

> We'll gain tremendous understanding of the basic, neurophysiological ways in which odors regulate the body and influence the mind … and we'll be able to influence behavior, modulate mood and alleviate pain.

Up-to-date scientific research has been set against primitive beliefs and traditions in an attempt to gain a more comprehensive understanding of the development and role of fragrance in our culture. Aromatherapy, which deals exclusively with natural botanical aromas, is at the forefront of this investigation, and there has even been a new term coined to describe this latest direction – 'psycho-aromatherapy'.

Psycho-aromatherapy refers to the practice of using natural aromatics specifically for their psychological effect. For this purpose, essential oils are utilized by means of vaporization, inhalation, baths, massage and in the form of a personalized 'perfume remedy' – the 'individual prescription'. The effect of the fragrance is thereby combined with other therapeutic techniques to maximize the psychological impact of the treatment. In this book, however, I have steered away from advocating particular oils for specific emotional complaints or for promoting a certain mood state. This is because it is impossible to accurately predict the effect of a given aroma without knowing the circumstances of the individual concerned. In the end result, our psychological response to fragrance is a highly personal phenomenon!

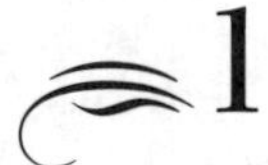

1

The Use of Aromatic Plants -Past, Present and Future

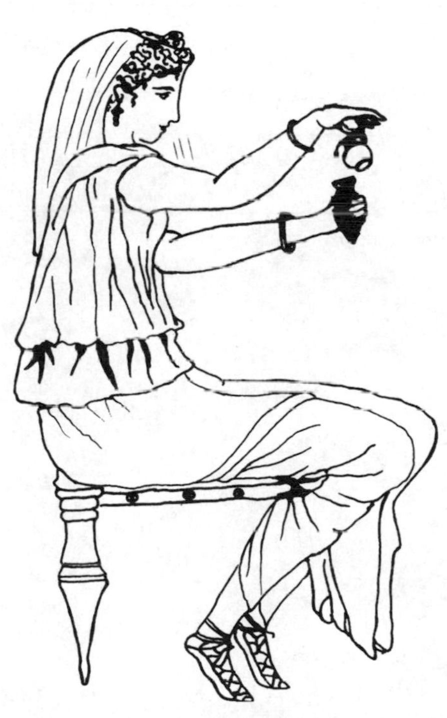

one 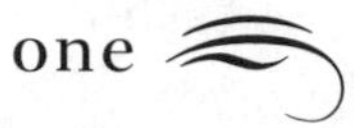

Aromatics: Medicine for the Mind

Where are they now, the days of aromatic warmth and hot-scented remedies!

Gaston Bachelard, *The Psychoanalysis of Fire*

In order to explore the role of aromatics and their effects on the mind, it is necessary to begin by first defining what is meant by 'mind', especially in its relation to the body. For unlike the physical organs and their functions, which can be described and understood in a straightforward manner, the mind by its very nature is much more subtle and difficult to grasp. This is made more complex by the fact that the definition of the word 'mind' has tended to vary in accordance with the cultural and philosophical attitudes of any given time or location. For the sake of simplicity, 'mind' is used here to denote anything of a psychological nature, including the emotional and spiritual disposition of an individual. Having said this, the very act of trying to isolate 'mind' from 'body' is based on false premises – in reality, the two are not separate entities, but rather interrelated aspects of a whole.

Medical attitudes regarding the relationship between the body and mind have also changed with the course of time. Theories concerning medical treatment have depended upon which aspect has been given pre-eminence within the cultural ethos of the society. Different cultures have at various times emphasized all aspects of the human condition – physical, emotional and spiritual – and have developed in diverse ways. In general, however, especially in the West, the evolution of ideas concerning the psyche-soma interaction can be seen to fall into three main epochs:

1) In the first, disease was thought to arise from causes external to the patient, never from 'natural causes' within the person. According to primitive belief, an illness was either caused by a malevolent spirit, sorcery on the part of an enemy or the evil influence of a deity. Sickness invoked by the transgression of some moral or religious law could only be remedied by a return to the correct mental or spiritual attitude. To be skilled in the practice of medicine in a primitive society therefore required an extensive knowledge of spells, charms and rituals – what we now call magic. The part played by psychological elements in this type of healing process was consequently of paramount importance.

2) In the second epoch, disease was regarded as the manifestation of an essentially physical or chemical imbalance, with secondary effects on the mind. The initial departure from the ancient magico-religious type of thinking can be traced to Hippocrates, known as the 'Father of Medicine'. He was the first to separate the practice of medicine from all religious or philosophical theory by focusing on the physical manifestation of the symptoms themselves. In establishing the method of 'clinical observation', he provided the foundation for the scientific approach that has dominated the medical field up to the present era.

3) In the third period, during which the term 'psychosomatic' has been introduced, an individual's well-being or ill-health are seen as 'anthropological' or involving the whole person. According to this view, the basis of all disease is a lack of wholeness. The cure is itself already implied by the words 'whole', 'holy', 'heal' and 'healthy', where health is not simply seen as an absence of illness but as a state of unity. This is the principle on which all 'holistic' therapies are based, including aromatherapy, where the overall aim is to bring the body and the mind into harmony through attention to the physical, emotional and spiritual needs.

Magic and Primitive Belief

> The sense of smell is the most important factor in the laying of spells on people: magic, in order to achieve the greatest potency, must enter through the nose.[1]

Psyche-soma interactions have preoccupied the human imagination since the dawn of civilization. The idea of a relationship between mankind and divinity, between matter and spirit, was one of the earliest forms of human conception. All primitive people embraced their own specific world-view, in which the role of man and woman in relation to their environment was expressed in terms of individual myths, legends or stories. Yet all these indigenous people shared a common understanding or belief: that we, as humans, are dependent upon maintaining a harmonious relationship between an external and an internal reality; between the seen and the unseen; between the body and the mind.

Life was understood as being dependent on a force which transcended the visible world, which was honoured by expression through specific rites and rituals. When an individual fell ill, it not only reflected an inner discord but also signified disharmony between that person and their environment with its governing forces. Fundamentally, disease was the manifestation of a state of disunity between the human realm and its supernatural agents. Consequently, in its earliest form, the art of healing was bound up with an ability to appease the spirit world, please the gods and combat curses.

Incense and aromatics played a significant role in such practices, since fragrant odours were thought to be favoured by the gods and many herbs were considered to have magical properties. Aromatics, medicine and magic consequently were very much interrelated in early cultures and the first physicians were invariably also priests, priestesses or shamans. As occult powers were thought to be sensitive to fragrant smoke or scents, a common way to cure a person sickened by the evil eye was to burn incense in the room. Among the Slavs, fumigation with aromatic plants was still being used until quite recently as a protection against epidemic fever, sorcery, witch bite or demonic charms. Amongst the herbs used for such purposes were sunflower, rue, pine, inula and garlic. The Australian aborigines still burn eucalyptus as a form of purification ritual to fumigate against sickness – 'heat went out of sick man and into fire'. Likewise, the Native Americans have preserved the ancient practice of burning aromatic plants like sage or cedarwood to produce a purifying smoke, which they call 'smudging'.

In North Africa, a newborn baby is protected from *djinns* or evil spirits by scented fumigations and with a balm made from saffron oil and henna. Similarly, before a marriage ceremony in North Africa can take place, the bride, who is particularly vulnerable to any jealous *djinn*, must undergo a whole series of purifications and perfumings. She also protects herself with incense and scented jewellery, especially a necklace made from tiny balls of saffron, orris, musk and benjamin.

The use of perfumed ornaments to appease the spirits is widespread in black Africa and throughout Asia. In India, the basil plant or *tulsi* is held to be holy, and its roots are made into sacred beads and rosaries. In Tibet, dry incense is worn as a talisman to ward off evil spirits and in Mexico a clove of garlic is still hung around the neck of a newborn as a protection. Amulets are commonly used in magical rites in all cultures and are often composed of, or include, aromatic materials.

Some herbs, such as rosemary, mugwort or St John's wort, have long been associated with magic or clairvoyant powers, and used as charms against evil. In Europe, a sprig of rosemary placed beneath the pillow was thought to protect the sleeper from nightmares, while a bunch of mugwort brought vivid dreams. A girdle of mugwort was also said to have been worn by John the Baptist in the wilderness, for it was used to ward off danger when travelling.

The odour of St John's wort was thought to drive away evil spirits, and it became a common custom to hang sprays of it above the doors of houses and churches on the eve of St John's Day, 24 June – the Summer Solstice, an ancient pagan festival.

> The possessed or insane were also obliged to inhale the odour of the crushed leaves and flowers, or drink a potion of it, in an effort to rid them of their madness.[2]

The origin of such measures was probably based on the inherent healing properties of the substance itself – St John's wort is recognized for its sedative and analgesic properties, and valued for combating hysterical conditions and 'menopausal neurosis'[3] for example, while garlic is now well known for its bactericidal and anti-infectious qualities. Many aromatic plants were ascribed special powers in this way based on direct experimentation, observation about the manner in which they grew, their healing potential and the effect of their fragrance. In Scandinavia, for instance, it was common until very recently to carry a lump of crude camphor as a protective measure during times of infectious illness, based on knowledge of its prophylactic powers.

However, the overall effectiveness of this type of ritual practice depends largely on the power of suggestion and the positive psychological attitude of the participants. One of the main premises underlying the magic art is the 'law of sympathy', i.e. the relationship between intention and manifestation, mind and matter. In this type of healing system, actions performed on a symbolic level in a ritual context are then brought about in actuality through a sympathetic response. Success is thus largely due to what in modern terminology is called the 'placebo effect'.

> In so far as these magic arts produce physiological and remedial effects, which they undoubtedly do, they might be classified under the head of psychic or mind medicine, the mental state aroused by a firm belief in their efficacy causing modifications of physiological function and even tissue change.[4]

The idea of healing through 'magic' or due to a 'placebo effect' tends to carry a negative connotation today – as if some kind of 'sham' or 'quackery' has taken place. Yet the power of belief has always been, and still is to a very large extent, a key factor in all healing systems (including modern allopathic medicine), and above all signifies the supremacy of mind over matter. Seen in this light, the cultivation of a positive mental attitude can be recognized as possibly the paramount factor in any healing process and consequently something to be emphasized rather then downgraded.

Ancient cultures considered that the psychological and spiritual disposition of a person was of vital importance to their well-being, not only as an individual but also with regard to their role within society. Restoration, achieved through the integration of individual and group, and the acknowledgement of a common causality for man and nature, was the foundation for all folk healing systems. Ill-health could not be treated simply through physical means – the specific mental and spiritual disposition of the individual also had to be taken into account. So herbs and aromatics were highly valued in these cultures not only as physical remedies but also for their positive psychic effects and rich symbolism.

Aromatic Remedies in Ancient Civilizations

> His nose he anoints and thinks it plain
> 'tis good for health with scents to feed the brain.[5]

The sacred dimension of the healing arts remained strong for thousands of years, as long as the interrelatedness of the body, mind and spirit was understood. Not only was this attitude dominant through the ancient civilizations of Mesopotamia, Egypt, Babylon and Greece, it was also prevalent in the Far East and in the West until the Middle Ages.

One of the earliest civilizations to develop a high degree of refinement was Mesopotamia, in the Near East around 3500 BC, whose most prominent city-state was Sumer. The Sumerian legacy to the healing arts has been especially profound and enduring. The oldest medical text in existence is recorded on two clay tablets from the Sumerian period.

Early Sumerian society was based on matriarchal principles, and the Mesopotamian goddess Ninlil was revered as protector of plants, crops, fertility, birth and death. Initially women had an important role in the healing arts and were included in all aspects of medical practice. There were two categories of practitioners: the *Ashipu* and the *Asu*. The former worked in the invisible or magical realm as a shamanic type of healer; the latter were versed in the botanical prescriptions used primarily to influence physical health. Aromatics featured largely in their culture and a clay pot that was possibly used for the distillation of plant essences has been found in a grave site dating back to 5500 BC. Gradually the Sumerians' knowledge and theories of medicine were carried via trade routes to the Phoenicians, Egyptians and Greeks. In this way, their civilization sent forth fingers of myth and culture into the surrounding regions which dominated the heritage of the Western world.

Egyptian medicine also dates back to prehistoric times and was supposed to have originated with the mythological deities of the country, notably Thoth, Osiris, Isis, Horus and Imhotep. It was practised largely by the priests and priestesses of these divinities, and consequently the preparation of remedies was generally accompanied by incantations and evocations. The ancient Egyptians were especially skilled in pharmacy, which is said to have been transmitted originally by the goddess Isis to her son Horus, who then communicated it to the priesthood. The 'Hermetic' medical books, having been given out by the god Thoth, came to be regarded as sacred, and any deviation from their rules as sacrilege. In the process of time, specialist healers developed who were knowledgeable about specific types of disease and their manner of treatment.

One of the earliest medical works on *materia medica*, pharmacy and therapeutics is the Egyptian Papyrus Ebers manuscript, discovered near Thebes in 1872. Written about 1552 BC in the time of Moses and before the exodus of the Israelites from Egypt, it contains numerous formulae for compounding various remedies and their methods of use. Saffron was employed as a condiment and perfume material; galbanum was used as an incense material; eagle wood was also used as an incense and for embalming the dead; cannabis or Indian hemp was used as a sedative and for its narcotic effect; mastic was much used for fumigation purposes, as were frankincense and myrtle.

Fumigation with fragrant herbs was one of the principal remedial and preventative measures in the treatment of disease used by the ancient Egyptians, Babylonians and Hebrews. Other aromatics which were common to all these cultures were myrrh, cumin, coriander, cyperus and balm of gilead.

Medicine was, however, still bound up with magical practices and most cures required a combination of physical remedies, spells and prayers. An ancient Babylonian tablet contains the following incantation for fever:

The sick man ... thou shalt place
... thou shalt cover his face
Burn cypress and herbs ...
That the great Gods may remove the evil
That the evil spirit may stand aside
... may a kindly spirit, a kindly genius be present.[6]

Spices and herbs were thus seen not only as physical remedies but also as 'charms' or 'magical drugs' which could influence the mental disposition of the patient and provide a mediating element through which a psychic healing could take place.

This was especially true of the ancient Greek cult of Asclepius. Like the Egyptian legacy, the primitive period of Greek medicine was part mythical, part historical. It begins with Melampus (*c.*1400 BC) and ends with Hippocrates (*c.*460 BC), but the most prominent figure during this period was Asclepius, reputed son of Apollo and Coronis. As the god of medicine he was worshipped by the Greeks and Romans alike, yet it is likely that his character was founded on that of an actual healer. The cult of Asclepius, which was centred around Epidaurus, combined magical or primitive therapeutic methods, such as the use of incantations, offerings and exorcisms, with an empirical approach, in which the overall psychological effect was considered paramount. Hundreds of temples were erected in Asclepius' honour and for many years priest-physicians, known as Asclepiades, practised a popular form of healing in these sanctuaries.

Central to their practice was a belief in the transformational relationship between the life-force and its housing – the body. The key to curing the body lay primarily in re-activating the primary life-force. Prayers and sacrifices were offered, and the sick were required to undergo a period of seclusion during which their dreams were recorded and interpreted by the priest-physicians. These were used as a means of insight into the cause and cure of the affliction, in much the same way as the traditional shaman sought out the roots of illness by assuming a trance state. Records of the cases, symptoms, treatment and results were carved upon votive tablets and hung upon the walls of the temples. The recipes for the therapeutic perfumes and incense which were used to enhance the psychological state of the patients are also recorded on some of these tablets. By the fourth century BC this type of healing had spread all over the Hellenic world and in some respects it was the forerunner of modern psycho-therapeutic practice.

Dioscorides (*c.* AD 100), the most renowned writer on *materia medica* of this period, mentions over 700 plants which were in use at the time and it may be assumed that they formed the basis of the remedies used in the temples of Asclepius with their focus on psychic medicine. In his *De Materia Medica*, a work which comprised the combined herbal lore of the Egyptians and Greeks, he discusses the components of perfumes and their medicinal properties, as well as listing detailed recipes. For example, he describes the perfume 'Susinum', as containing cardamom, cinnamon, lilies, myrrh, saffron, balanus, wine and honey. Among other aromatics mentioned are: absinthe, anise, balm, basil, calamus, chenopodium, clove, coriander, cumin, fennel, frankincense, galbanum, garlic, hyssop, juniper, laurel, marjoram, melilot, mint, mugwort, myrtle, narcissus, nard, origanum, pennyroyal, pepper, pine, rock rose (labdanum), rose, rosemary, rue, sage, styrax, tarragon, thuja, thyme, turpentine, verbena, violet and wormwood.

However, the most extensive literary information about the early therapeutic use of aromatics and their effect on the mind comes from the classical writer, Theophrastus (*c*.300 BC). In his *Enquiry into Plants*, Theophrastus describes the properties of various oils and spices and explores the qualities of the odours themselves. He mentions specific herbs which affect the mental powers: two varieties of a plant known as *strykhnos* (a type of thorn apple), one which upsets the mental powers and 'makes one mad' and another which induces sleep. He also mentions the root of *onotheras* (oleander) which, when administered in wine, makes the 'temper gentler and more cheerful'.

In ancient Greece, physicians who cured through the use of 'aromatic unctions' were known as *Iatralypte*. Scented ointments and oils were recognized as having great benefit on both the physical and psychological level. Bay laurel was used to produce a trance-like state, and roses, costus, myrtle and coriander had aphrodisiac properties, while myrrh and marjoram were considered soporific. The Greek physicians adopted many of the Egyptian perfume/remedy formulations, including 'The Egyptian' and 'Kyphi' – which were said to cure by 'transfer of sympathy'. A substance such as 'Kyphi', which contained 16 different ingredients, could be used as a perfume, an incense or a medicine. It was said to be anti-septic, balsamic and an antidote to poison which, according to Plutarch, would 'lull one to sleep, allay anxiety and brighten dreams ... made of those things that delight most in the night'.[7]

Another such drug was the miraculous drug *nepenthe*, described in *The Odyssey*, that Helen of Troy (*c.* 2000 BC) is supposed to have obtained from Egypt. The drug has been the subject of much controversy – opinion varies as to whether it was concocted from opium, datura, cannabis, evening primrose or verbena and adiantum mixed:

> And now she dropped into the wine they were drinking
> a drug – an anodyne, bile-allaying, causing one to forget all ills ...[8]

Helen and the other Homeric heroes and heroines had a credible pharmacopoeia, particularly for relieving pain and altering moods. Mention is made of hellebore, mandrake and poppy juice, inhaled from a steaming sponge. Poppy (later purified opium) was used as an anaesthetic, belladonna and mandrake as anti-spasmodics, cannabis as a euphoric and in the treatment of bronchitis. Myrrh also had its uses – added to wine, it comforted the mind and produced a trance-like state. This property was later utilized by a group of Jewish women known as 'The Daughters of Jerusalem', who offered victims due to be crucified a wine in which myrrh had been dissolved, to help relieve the pain. Frankincense dissolved in wine was also used as a general anaesthetic.

The Mind/Body Split

Yet, it is with the Greeks that the first signs of a division between the mind and the body, the human and natural realm, became apparent. This development heralded the abandonment of 'magical medicine' in favour of 'scientific materialism'. In his book *The Return of the Goddess*, E. Whitmont traces the evolution of consciousness from the magical, through the mythological to the mental phase – the age of reason.

> The mythological phase of consciousness is a bridge from magical to mental functioning. As the hot lava of the magical level is touched by the first, cold air of the discerning mind, it gels into forms ... It marks the transition from a gynolatric to an androlatric world and reaches back to the cult of the Goddess and her child consort who constantly dies and is reborn.[9]

In the magical and early mythological phase, dominated by worship of the Goddess, everything was seen as partaking of *mana*, everything was seen as sacred. Aromatics, with their inherent connection to the magical, non-material aspects of existence, were throughout this period regarded as valuable tools of transformation. But as rational, patriarchal consciousness gained the ascendancy, the non-rational, intuitive feminine principle was relegated, as was the woman's role in healing. Subduing the passions meant repressing the feminine aspect and upholding the masculine ideal of 'self-control'. Since odour provided a direct doorway through to the feminine part of the mind, the non-rational or 'magical' domain, the ancient preoccupation with aromatics as 'mind-medicine' also began to wane.

Hippocrates, the son of a priest-physician of Asclepius, was the first to formulate a new approach to medical practice. He separated medicine from priestcraft by maintaining that disease was not due to possession by evil spirits or the like, but to an imbalance of fluid matter related to internal, emotional and external factors. He developed a new theory of disease based on the four elements and the four humours. According to his theory, earth was associated with black bile, air with yellow bile, fire with blood and water with phlegm. One's temperament and constitution were dependent upon the balance of these qualities. If the body was too cold and dry, for example, it indicated an excess of black bile, so there would be a tendency towards melancholy.

But just as physical illness could be seen to affect the mind, so stress and powerful emotions could influence the body and its behaviour:

> Fears, shame, pain, pleasure, passion and so forth: to each of these an appropriate member of the body responds by its action. Instances are sweats, palpitation of the heart, and so forth.[10]

Hippocrates recognized a psychosomatic unity in mental and physical diseases, for he wrote: 'In order to cure the human body it is necessary to have knowledge of the whole.'[11] As part of his treatment, he prescribed aromatics, such as the famous *megalion*, made from myrrh, cinnamon and cassia, which, like the Egyptian 'Kyphi', functioned both as a physical remedy and as a mentally reviving elixir. He also maintained that the key to good health rested on having a daily aromatic bath and a scented massage. However, although Hippocrates and the other great minds of his time drew extensively on the wisdom of Mesopotamia, Egypt and Babylon as well as the other great medical traditions of the East, disease was now regarded primarily as arising from natural causes which could be located in the physical body.

Following Hippocrates' scientific method, Galen (AD 130–200) described disorders in terms of warmth, cold, dryness and moisture, and erected the foundations of modern physiology. All diseases, mental as well as physical, were, according to Galen, due to a disorder of the humours. He was disdainful of the magical element inherent in Egyptian healing methods and wrote disapproving of the ' ... silly Egyptian spells with incantations, which the Egyptians utter while picking their herbal drugs ...'.[12]

That this development took place at the expense of sacrificing the psychological aspect was recognized by Socrates, when he quoted the Thracian king Zamolxis's views on treatment:

> ... as you ought not to attempt to cure the eyes without the head, or the head without the body, so neither ought you to attempt to cure the body without the soul; and that is the reason why the cure of many diseases is unknown to the physicians of Hellas.[13]

Nevertheless, herbal remedies still constituted the main materials at the physicians' disposal, and aromatic plants and essences were still used widely. Fragrant oils were commonly used for basic hygiene, especially when water was scarce and soap non-existent. Evidence from Egypt, Greece, Rome and the Near East indicates that both men and women oiled their skin as well as their hair with fragrant lotions to prevent dryness and keep the skin supple, while perfumes were used to mask less pleasant odours. Homer frequently mentions oils being applied after a bath or instead of one! Scent was still considered to be the most effective way of cleansing polluted air, and bonfires of scented wood and flowers permeated with perfumed unguents were lit in the streets of Athens during times of plague.

Aromatics were also still valued for their soothing or stimulating properties. The Greeks described the scent of hyacinth as being uplifting and invigorating to a tired mind, and Galen considered the fragrance of narcissus oil to be 'the food of the soul'. In the Greek world, the need to take care of the body was also to a great extent connected with sport. During the great games at Daphne, the Greek king employed 200 girls to sprinkle rosewater on the crowd to refresh their spirits. Before a competition, the athletes would oil their skin and sprinkle it with a powder appropriate to the type of sport they were doing. In private houses too, anointing the body with oil was a routine matter for maintaining health and beauty.

Perfume also played a central role in the Roman ritual of bathing. It was employed in three principal modes: solid unguents (*hedysmata*) – generally a single scent such as almond, rose or quince; liquid unguents (*stymmata*) – compounded perfumes containing flowers, spices and gums; or powder perfumes (*diapasmata*) – pulverised aromatics. Thus incense and perfumes continued to be used in lavish quantities both for pleasure and for the effect they had on the mind and spirit.

The Christian Legacy

> Christian theology forged an absolute gulf between humanity and nature. Pagan worship of the divinity within nature was rejected.[14]

Under the Romans, however, as the papacy grew in strength, the Church became increasingly sensitive to any competition from physicians with regard to the cure of the mind or soul. The third century AD also witnessed a rapidly shrinking market for myrrh and frankincense, due to the opposition of the early puritanical Christians to what they saw as 'pagan fragrances'. In their eyes, the human body and its natural instincts were something to be regarded with distrust and repulsion and, since perfumes and incense stimulated the senses and could be used to heighten sensual pleasure, they were rejected by the Church.

Then in AD 529 Pope Gregory the Great passed a decree that forbade any form of learning that was not acceptable to the political ambitions of the papacy. This included knowledge of *materia medica*. The School of Philosophy at Athens was closed the same year and the works of Galen and Hippocrates had to be smuggled to Syria.

Arab physicians played an important role in the development of medicine, especially with regard to the prophylactic and therapeutic use of odours. By the third century AD, Alexandria was a vital centre and repository for Greek science and the Alexandrian School of Chemists was developing the process of distillation. Later, Avicenna (AD 980–1037) improved upon this process by inventing the apparatus and method of alembic distillation for the extraction of essential oils. He did much to promote the benefits of aromatic oils and their life-giving virtues:

> For the Prophet ... the interest in using excellent odours is that they fortify the senses. And when the senses are strong, the thoughts are strong and the conclusions upright. When, on the other hand, the senses become weak, thoughts become unbalanced and their conclusions confused.[15]

The convergence between ancient ideas and contemporary Arab concepts influenced physicians to use essential oils increasingly for their purifying, restorative and reviving capabilities. Aromatics were back in vogue! They were thought to combat the organism's destructive passions like fear and sorrow which make the body more susceptible to illness. Being surrounded by pleasant odours was consequently seen as a way of ensuring good health and preventing the spread of disease, especially during times of plague.

By the thirteenth century, 'the perfumes of Arabia' and the therapeutic use of aromatic oils had spread throughout Europe. In France during the 1348 plague, the Collegium of the Faculté de Paris prescribed the 'cold' scent of roses, sandalwood, nenuphar and camphor during the summertime, and hot aromatics like eagle wood, amber, nutmeg, sweet gum or 'pomander' during the winter months. Pomanders, which originated in the East, were hollow spheres of ornamental gold or silver containing solid perfumes which only the rich could afford, such as musk, aloes, cinnamon and ambergris. In Britain during the Middle Ages, pomanders, scent boxes and 'tussie mussies' (little posies of aromatic herbs) were popular, while the floors of dwelling-places were strewn with sweet rushes, rose petals, lemon leaves, chamomile and other herbs.

In the minds of the common people however, perfumes were still bound up with magic and superstition. In the Anglo-Saxon *Leech Book of Bald*, a sprig of rosemary was recommended as a protection against evil spirits, while in the thirteenth-century *Myddfai* manuscripts, it says of the same herb:

> If the leaves be put beneath your pillow, you will be well protected from troublesome dreams and all mental anxiety.[16]

After the Protestant reformation of 1517, the employment of aromatics and incense in Britain was again reduced by the Church – only the Roman Catholic Church, with its emphasis on the symbolic value of ritual, retained their use. Seventeenth-century spirituality further strengthened the contempt for the senses and the physical body. The founder of the Order of Redemptorists laid great stress on olfactory mortification:

> As for the sense of smell, do not be so vain as to surround yourselves with amber perfumes and other sweet smelling compounds or to use toilet water, all of which have little to recommend them, even to the laity.[17]

The devaluation of the senses and their effect on the emotions was furthered by the philosophical climate as well as by ecclesiastical principles. René Descartes (1596–1650) defined man's body as a machine with the soul located in the pineal gland at the base of the brain and to John Locke (1632–1704), who saw all knowledge as built up from bodily sensation, emotion was purely physiological. For the healing arts, the direction given by Descartes' work was a turning-point – mind and body were conceived as having no relationship to one another, and the concept of 'soul' was eroded.

Throughout the eighteenth and early nineteenth centuries, the emotions were given a visceral location, though controversy became acute at this time over whether disorders of the mind brought about physical changes in the body or whether physical disease upset the mind. In 1763, the physician Gaub wrote a response to Julien La Mettries' essay 'Man, a Machine', which he summarized in the following way:

> 1) The causes and occasions of a great many affections of the body arise in the mind.
> 2) The mind can be a bulwark of health.
> 3) In many cases of bodily disease treatment must be directed against the mind as the source of the bodily complaint.

> 4) Bodily diseases may often be more readily alleviated or cured by the mind, that is, by the emotions, than by 'corporeal remedies'.[18]

Gaub recommended that physicians should actively search for substances capable of affecting the mind and that it would be a 'happy and fruitful endeavour for some far-sighted persons to occupy themselves with a subject of such importance'.[19] One such 'far-sighted person' was Charles Fourier, an ardent defender of the emotions, who even as a child dreamt of subjecting 'aromas' to true scientific study. He set about cultivating a wide selection of aromatic species and conducted a series of personal experiments on the effects of their fragrance. He believed that perfumes, being linked to the powers of attraction or aversion, pleasure or repulsion, served to 'guide men and beasts' on an instinctual level. Apart from its profound influence on the human and animal passions, he saw scent as being fundamental to all existence.

Fourier's notion of a cosmic olfactory foundation to all of life was to anticipate the results of contemporary astrophysicists by nearly 200 years. Results of the recent *Arome* experiment carried out by the French National Centre for Scientific Research include one highly important discovery:

> It has been found that aromatic molecules are one of the basic components of the interstellar space in which new stars are constantly being formed. This interstellar 'atmosphere' or gas is the almost direct source of the atoms of which we ourselves, along with the earth and the other planets, are made.[20]

A Modern Marriage

Human consciousness has moved forward and the individual perception of the universe is very different today from that of 6,000 years ago. It is fruitless simply to try and return to the primitive magico-religious approach to healing methods in an attempt to compensate for the materialistic approach of the previous era. Yet some type of integration is required and looking towards the East can perhaps provide an inspiration. Some of the oriental traditions, such as the Indian, Chinese and Tibetan medical systems, have not suffered from the same mind/body split as has the Western approach:

> … where the Greeks were ready to apportion separate spheres of influence to the natural and the supernatural, and therefore created the terrain in which a strictly material interpretation of disease could grow, Hindu Philosophy kept the two spheres closely intermingled, giving rise to a medical system in which non-material aspects could have as much, if not more, influence than material ones.[21]

The Indian medical system, which has its origins in the magico-religious vision of the Vedic literature, has evolved into a sophisticated evolutionary classification of matter and spirit based on Hindu philosophy. Life is regarded as the mutual interaction of body, mind and soul, where the mediating factor is the life-force or *prana* (in Chinese *chi*). According to this system, there are two primary principles, known as *purusa* and *prakrti* (similar to the Chinese *yin–yang* system). The former is passive and connected with the spirit; the latter is active and represents primordial matter, which in turn gives rise to *sattva*, *rajas* and *tamas* – the essence of thought, energy and matter. Indian medicine is consequently divided into three parts: *Unani*, which uses prayer and invocation; *Sidhata*, which includes knowledge of the chakras, the means for the transformation of energy within the individual; and *Ayurveda*, which is the knowledge and use of medicinal plants for healing purposes. In *Ayurvedic* medicine, a form of aromatherapy has been practised as one element of holistic treatment for thousands of years. Many aromatic plants are included in the making of medicinal oils for massage, or mixed with wine or honey as internal remedies.

Since aromatic essences also contain the life-force of a plant, they can help re-activate or harmonize the *prana* or *chi* within an individual, which is vital to the overall healing process.

Some remedies, on the other hand, are most effective in the form of an incense, fumigant or inhalation, especially for the treatment of psychological disorders.

The Tibetan remedy 'Aquilaria A' contains 31 ingredients, including eagle wood, clove, cardamom, myrrh, sandalwood and nutmeg, and its inhalation is especially recommended for insomnia, anxiety, tension, hysteria and other psychological symptoms. Like the Indian approach, the Tibetan view of medicine is that a permanent cure can only take place when spiritual, emotional and physical factors are in harmony. A physician's prescription can consequently include advice on specific spiritual or ritual practices, as well as the administration of physical remedies.

The Western approach to medicine is beginning to change. Current attitudes reflect the growing recognition that disease is psychosomatic in nature and that it is not enough to treat a person simply on a physical or chemical basis – the individual as a whole needs to be taken into account. The twentieth century has seen an enormous growth in holistic forms of medicine and a vast increase in the use of natural remedies. Many ancient forms of therapy are enjoying a revival, but in a modern form – including aromatherapy. For although the term 'aromatherapy' is new, the practice itself is founded on a system which has been in use for thousands of years. When the French perfumer René Gattefossé published his book *Aromathérapie* in the 1920s, describing the physical and psychological benefits of using natural aromatics, particularly essential oils, in therapeutic practice, he was simply reviving and updating an ancient healing system. In contemporary aromatherapy, we are in fact witnessing a marriage of the traditional and the modern, the spiritual and the scientific, although the integration is by no means complete. The conflict between 'orthodox' and 'alternative' types of treatment is still being fought, as Western medicine struggles to find a more balanced perspective.

> One point is clear; in the present century the importance of the person has reached a new phase … To realize that the patient is a personal as well as a chemical and physical entity is to realize that disease may arise at a personal level; that health consists of an harmonious blend of human physics and chemistry with emotional urges.[22]

In recent years James Lovelock has popularized the Gaia principle, named after the Greek goddess of the earth. According to this theory, our whole planet is itself a living being with its own spirit or intelligence, in which all of existence participates. This new approach, which reconnects humanity with nature and re-endows matter with consciousness, heralds a return to the primitive yet transformed principle of an inherent sacredness or spirituality within the universe. It is significant that the latest advances in biochemistry and molecular physics also corroborate this vision – that of a universal 'mind' or 'consciousness' which transcends space or time:

> Paradoxically, this new dimension of mind is also what reconnects each of these sciences to their ancient roots before there was a division between mind/spirit and matter. On a fundamental level, this is what aromachology and psycho-aromatherapy are really about, the reintegration of mind and fragrance.[23]

References

1. Malinowski, 1929, cited in Schleidt, M., 'The Semiotic Relevance of Human Olfaction' in Dodd, G. H. and Van Toller, S., *Fragrance: The Psychology and Biology of Perfume II*, Elsevier Science Publications Ltd., 1992, p.47.
2. le Strange, R., *A History of Herbal Plants*, Angus and Robertson, 1977, p.47.
3. *British Herbal Pharmacopoeia*, British Herbal Medicine Association, 1983, p.115.
4. Whitebread, C., *The Magic, Psychic, Ancient Egyptian, Greek and Roman Medical Collections*, US National Museum, p.3.
5. Alexis.
6. An ancient Babylonian tablet, cited in Tisserand, R., *The Art of Aromatherapy*, C. W. Daniel, 1985, p.20.
7. Plutarch.
8. Homer, *The Odyssey*, IV, pp.220–32.
9. Whitmont, E. C., *The Return of the Goddess*, Routledge and Kegan Paul, 1983, p.49.
10. Hippocrates, *Humours*, cited in Castrén, P., *Ancient and Popular Healing*, Vammalan Kirjapaino Oy, Vammala, 1989, p.91.
11. Ibid.
12. Galen, *De simlicium medicamentorum temperamentis ac facultatibus* 6, XI, p.792.
13. Socrates, cited in Poynter & Keele, *A Short History of Medicine*, Mills and Boon, 1961, p.66.
14. Whitmont, p.98.
15. Cited in Le Guérer, A., *Scent: The Mysterious Power of Smell*, Chatto and Windus, 1993, p.66.
16. Cited in Conway, D., *The Magic of Herbs*, Mayflower, 1973, p.136.
17. Alphonse Marie de Liguori, *The True Spouse of Jesus Christ*, cited in Le Guérer, A., op. cit., p.163.
18. Cited in Rather, L. J., *Mind and Body in 18th Century Medicine*, Wellcome Historical Medical Library, 1965, p.195.
19. Ibid., p.113.
20. Omont, Alain, 'Les molecules aromatiques de milieu interstellaire' in *Aux Frontières de la Science, La Recherche*, 1989, p.XXXVI.

21. Bellamy, D. and Pfister, A., *World Medicine,* Blackwell, 1992, p.46.
22. Poynter and Keele, *A Short History of Medicine,* Mills and Boon, 1961, p.46.
23. Steele, J., 'In Profile' in *The International Journal of Aromatherapy*, vol.5, no.1, 1993, p.9.

two 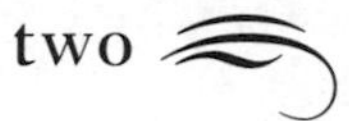

The Ritual Use of Incense

The fire is laid, the fire shines;
The incense is laid on the fire, the incense shines.
Your perfume comes to me, O Incense;
May my perfume come to you, O Incense.
Your perfume comes to me, you Gods;
May my perfume come to you, you Gods.
May I be with you, you Gods;
May you be with me, you Gods …

Utterance 269, Pyramid Texts[1]

The term 'incense' has been used in a variety of different ways throughout history. In its widest sense, it refers to a material which emits fragrant fumes by burning or vaporization. Often it indicates 'smoke', but it also implies 'odour'. In ancient times incense was either composed of a single aromatic substance, notably frankincense, or was compounded of a variety of essential oils, gums, resins and spices. These were usually thrown on a fire in the form of a powder or granules, sprinkled on lighted charcoal to be offered upon an incense altar, or put inside an incense burner or censer, which could be held in the hand. Alternatively, the incense material was mixed with vegetable oils and possibly other ingredients such as honey, wax or fat and shaped into balls or cones which melted when exposed to heat, or applied to a person or the image of a deity directly in the form of an 'unguent' or oily perfume. In ancient times, there was in fact little distinction between incense and perfume. Indeed, the word 'perfume' is derived from the Latin *per fumen*, meaning 'to smoke'. Any real difference between the two only developed, at least with regard to ingredients, as late as the fourteenth century in the West with the discovery of new alcoholic extraction techniques.

Communication with the Divine

Aromatics have been used as offerings and as a means of communication with the divine from time immemorial. The archaeological records and remains which have survived over thousands of years inform us that all the early civilizations used incense for worship, and that the burning of aromatic plants and oils played a central role in their cultures, especially with regard to their religious customs.

The earliest recorded use of incense comes from ancient China, though few details of the actual rites have survived. It is probable that the Hindus absorbed the cult of incense from the Chinese and opened up the first trading routes to the incense lands of Arabia as well as to Egypt around 3600 BC.

The Sumerians and Babylonians burned incense as a means of purification and to please their gods, while to the Hebrews the smoke of incense veiled the presence of the deity in the holy tabernacle. The early Persians used incense in their worship, as depicted on the monuments at Persepolis, and Muslims still frequently offer incense in the shrines of their saints today. The Greeks and Romans, especially the latter, were lavish in their use of incense and frankincense is still used in the Roman Catholic Church in the West. The Native Americans used fumigation as part of their ritual practices, as did many other indigenous races, such as the Australian aborigines. Even in early America, the Mayas of Mexico burned balls of copal incense for their gods and used perfume as an integral part of their grotesque practice of human sacrifice:

> Blood and incense seem fated by nature to fulfil an identical function – to establish communication with the divine.[2]

Egyptian Practices

The ancient Egyptians were renowned for their knowledge and expertise regarding aromatics, and the use of incense in Egypt goes back to prehistoric times. It was from Egypt and the Mesopotamian basin in the Near East that the earliest tangible evidence in the form of aromatic remnants and cult objects have emerged. Resin balls have been found in several predynastic tombs and resinous materials continue to occur among the grave treasures of dynastic times. Balls of incense were discovered in Tutankhamun's tomb.

Already at the time of the Old Kingdom (2686–2181 BC) the preparation and specific purposes of incense had been established. The ingredients and manufacture of various scents have been preserved on temple walls, together with directions for their use. The recipe for 'Kyphi', for example, is shown on the inner temple walls at Edfu, within the sacred precinct of the temple priests. This precious perfume and incense was made from a mixture of over 16 aromatic substances including juniper, cardamom, calamus, cyperus (a fragrant grass), matic, saffron, acacia, henna, cinnamon, peppermint and myrrh, blended into a paste containing over 25 per cent resin, then shaped into pellets to be burned on specific occasions.

Indeed, incense was indispensable for all aspects of ancient Egyptian ritual practice, notably for the elaborate ceremonies surrounding death. During the funeral rites of a dead king, incense and aromatics were not only used to protect the physical corpse from decay and to disguise the stench of putrefaction, but also to confer the transformation from the human state to that of a divinity. In *The Book of the Dead*, incense is called for in many rites to purify and protect the soul in the after-life, and to ensure a safe passage.

> From the Pyramid Texts, we learn that there is a purificatory use of incense in that the King is purified from all evil odours, an apotropaic use of incense in that incense is able to protect him from evil, and what may be called a mediatory use of incense in the sense that incense is used as a means of establishing contact between man and god, a contact which can bring man to heaven or god to earth.[3]

Incense was thus used to bring the human and transcendent worlds closer together – the ascending smoke was seen symbolically as a vehicle by which prayers could be carried to the deities above and as a means of communication between the two realms. What does this mean in modern psychological language? It suggests that scent has the power to evoke our highest aspirations and fears, and can be used to transport us onto another plane of consciousness.

The invisible yet influential effect of odour was well known to the ancient Egyptians who utilized its remarkable power: the ability to penetrate the unseen realms of the psyche and affect the inner dimensions of the mind. 'Kyphi' for example, was burned on ritual occasions to heighten the senses and spiritual awareness of the priests, and to raise the spirits of their 'congregation'.

According to the ancient Egyptian world-view, the human realm was governed by a resident deity, sustained through offerings from the king or, in his absence, the high priests. The image of the deity was tended daily – washed, censed, anointed, clothed and fed – and in return the god ensured the equilibrium and good fortune of the people. According to myth, several of the deities were themselves associated with various aromatics – Nefertum, the god of perfumers, incense and fragrant oils, was identified with the sacred blue lotus, while his consort Sekhmet, the goddess of healing and alchemy, was known as the 'lady of every herb'. Myrrh was derived from the tears of the god Horus, while plants used for incense were produced from the tears of Shu and Tefnut.

The early Egyptians also believed that their deities were nourished by odours and incense was commonly thought to be 'the food of the Gods'. The 'Ka', or double of the body, which resided in sacred statues and in the mummy, took pleasure in scents, while its 'Ba', or soul, actually fed on incense and offerings. Since scent delighted the human senses, it was naturally assumed that the deities found it especially pleasing. By burning aromatics the Egyptians believed they could ensure divine favour and attract special attention to their prayers. In many temple murals the king himself can be seen standing before the statue of a god holding a smoking censer in his hands.

At Heliopolis, the City of the Sun, incense was burned in the temple three times a day in honour of the sun-god Ra: in the morning with gum arabic; at midday with myrrh; and at sunset with 'Kyphi'. The nightly offering of 'Kyphi' ensured the return of the sun the following morning! Incense and libations were also offered during the coronation ceremony, to celebrate a military victory and before the opening of a shrine containing a deity.

The two main types of aromatics used by the ancient Egyptians were known as *ntyw* and *sntr*. The former most probably referred to myrrh (bdellium/sweet myrrh) which was also used in the form of *stacte* – oil of myrrh. *Ntyw*, which was employed in perfumes, medicines and cosmetics as well as incense, was the product *par excellence* imported from the 'Land of Punt', i.e. Somalia on the north African coast. *Sntr*, meaning 'God's odour', was also imported in smaller quantities from Punt and most probably referred to a variety of frankincense – either *Boswellia carteri*, *B. frerenan* or *B. papyrifera*. It was used exclusively as an incense, though inferior in quality to the true sacred incense *B. sacra*, which is only found in southern Arabia. An expedition to the Land of Punt depicted on a temple relief shows Queen Hatshepsut receiving a ship loaded with vast quantities of aromatics brought back from the 'incense terraces'. Expeditions to Punt were recorded as early as 2800 BC under the patronage of King Sahure. It was only around the first century AD that the focus of the incense trade swung towards Arabia.

The Near East

At about the same time as the birth of Jesus, incense materials were being brought overland to Egypt by Arabian traders. The best type of frankincense (*B. sacra*) grew in southern Arabia and its high value was matched only by myrrh and gold, which together represented the three costliest commodities of the ancient world – suitable gifts for a newborn king! The 'perfumes of Arabia' also constituted some of the earliest trade items between East and West. Pliny reported that the southern Arabian kingdoms of Hadramout and Dhofar were the wealthiest states in the world because of their monopoly of the frankincense trade, yet little is known about the exact ritual practices of the early Arabian civilization. They certainly used aromatic resins and gums extensively in their religious practices and erected specific incense altars within their temples. These small cube-shaped altars, which often stood on four short legs, were made from limestone, terracotta or clay and were decorated with regular geometric designs. The names of various aromatics were inscribed on the sides of the altars – some had many names, some only one. Frankincense, myrrh, storax and mastic occur quite frequently, being indigenous to the area. Spikenard and costus are also among those mentioned – these were probably imported from India. On some altars, the burnt remains of incense are still discernible in their basins thousands of years later. Incense burners were also often placed in tombs.

Another trade route from southern Arabia went eastward towards Syria–Mesopotamia. Like the Egyptians, the Assyro-Babylonians required vast quantities of aromatics for use in their rituals. They gathered them from the richly forested Amanus mountains in Syria or imported them from Arabia. The wood, resin or sap of a wide variety of aromatic substances, including myrtle, galbanum, tamarisk, cypress, bdellium, cedar, frankincense, ladanum, spikenard, myrrh, calamus, mastic, juniper and opobalsam, were used as incense in ancient Syria and Mesopotamia. The incense was offered either upon an incense altar, similar to those found in southern Arabia; on a hollow pottery shrine, specimens of which have been traced to the third millennium BC;4 in an incense 'lamp' designed to hook on the wall; in a vase-shaped censer; or in a shallow bowl placed on top of a tall cylindrical pottery stand, which is depicted in many Assyrian relief carvings. These often contain a conical mound of incense which looks very similar to the cones of incense or 'unguent' used by the Egyptians, which were composed of a blend of powders, oils, resins and fats.

Like the early Egyptian term for 'perfume', the Mesopotamian word for 'unguent' had religious associations. Assyrian sculptures at Ninevah show incense being burned for the sun-god and it is known that the Assyrians used aromatics during rituals connected with the cult of the dead. The Babylonians also sometimes sprinkled their meat offerings with incense as a way of consecrating the food, making it holy and therefore acceptable to the gods.

But again, the principal and underlying basis for the use of incense in Syria and Mesopotamia was the belief that its odour ensured divine favour. Where incense was burned, the gods assembled – as if they actually manifested their presence through scent. It was also thought that the fragrance of the incense worked like a drug on the minds of the gods, as well as on the minds of men: their wrath was calmed, they gave positive oracles (incense smoke was used as a form of divination) and looked kindly on the misdeeds of man. Incense was the means by which the human soul could be cleansed before the face of god:

> Incense, dwelling in the mountain, created in the mountains,
> you are pure coming from the mountains.

Fragrance of juniper, fragrance of cedar, incense dwelling in the mountains.
The powerful incense has been granted to us,
the high mountains provide it for purification
in the pure censer, filled with awe inspiring splendor,
the sweet oil, the choice oil, worthy of the table,
and the pure [aromatics], the materials of the purifying craft.

Make the incense fumes, their purifying product, issue forth:
May he be clean like heaven, may he be pure like the core of heaven,
may the evil tongue stand aside![5]

It is clear from this text that to the Assyro-Babylonians incense was also a substance of purification, especially with regard to those rich odoriferous resins derived from coniferous trees like cedar, juniper and cypress. This corresponds to the central idea behind many Oriental practices, especially those of the Buddhists, in which incense is used extensively as a means of purification.

The Far East

The Chinese have one of the most ancient systems of herbal medicine, which includes a vast number of indigenous species, such as the Chinese or Japanese angelica, but also imported aromatics. Sandalwood, for example, is listed as an incense and medicine in numerous ancient Chinese texts. Apart from sandalwood, the Chinese have also used storax and the powdered bark of cinnamon and cassia as incense from very early times. Balls of jasmine were used in China to cleanse the atmosphere surrounding the sick and to scent the air during public festivals. Bronze incense burners found in China date back to the Shang Dynasty (1600–1030 BC) and incense still forms an essential element in the religious ceremonies of the Far East today. Borneo camphor, for example, has been used as an incense in the East since ancient times and is still burned in China at funerals.

Like China, India has always been very rich in herbal plants and aromatics have played an important role in traditional medicinal practices as well as religious rituals for thousands of years. The Hindus adopted the ritual use of incense from the Chinese and introduced other ingredients, including frankincense, sarsaparilla seeds, benzoin and cyprus into the recipe. They were the first to use the roots of plants, such as that of the lime tree (*Tilia*) and Indian spikenard as incense materials. Strongly scented floral fragrances, such as jasmine or rose, also contribute to the characteristic sweetish scent of Indian incense. Fragrances like saffron, cassia, cardamom, cinnamon, aloe-wood, basil and patchouli are also common. In Hindu temples, the god Shiva is offered incense every four hours, mainly frankincense and cyprus.

However, the most popular incense material throughout the Far East is derived from the sandalwood tree. The highest quality comes from Mysore in eastern India. In India the oil is often combined with rose in the famous perfume *aytar*, which is used to purify body and soul. Sandalwood, cloves, cardamom and curcuma are also blended to form a powder called *abir* which is used during Hindu ceremonies. In Tantric yoga, sandalwood is described as the scent of the 'subtle body', and is used to awaken the *kundalini* energy and transform it into enlightenment.

Other early evidence of aromatic materials used for ritual purposes in the Far East has been found in the Indus Valley, at the foot of the Himalayas. Harrappan figures of the Mother Goddess dated to the third millennium BC still show the dark stains left by incense smoke. Thousands of years later in Tibet and Nepal, incense is still in use as an offering and purification material, as exemplified by the Tibetan Buddhist *Riwo Sangcho* or 'Smoke Puja'. During the rite, cypress and juniper – 'incense offering of the mountains' – is commonly burned in order to purify all past *karma*, and combat and appease negative influences including 'the elementals who cause disease and bring obstacles, the evil portents of dreams and all kinds of bad omen'.[6] This Tibetan rite typically combines animistic-type beliefs with later Buddhist concepts, which ultimately transforms the practice from a purely personal ritual into one which embraces the whole of existence.

Incense was introduced to Japan together with Buddhism in AD 538. For the following 200 years it was used exclusively on Buddhist altars, before being gradually integrated into the everyday life of the Japanese people. Over the next few centuries the practice of scenting clothes using a censer containing resinous balls of incense became extremely popular and aristocrats are known to have fumigated their rooms with a variety of aromatics. At this time, all the incense materials used in Japan were imported via China from different parts of the world. Prominent among the substances used were sandalwood, camphor, borneol, cassia, costus, spikenard, tumeric, angelica, clove, styrax, benzoin, frankincense and aloe or eagle wood.

By the eleventh century, the art of combining different scents had developed into the 'incense competition', where interested parties got together to try and guess the composition of their fellow-contestants' compounds. At the same time, the art of 'listening' to incense became associated with the aesthetic appreciation of the period, where a judge would comment on each recipe and express in poetic form the type of mood evoked by its form and fragrance.

Then in the fifteenth century, the 'kodo ceremony' or 'art of incense' was born. Like the tea ceremony, which emerged during the same epoch, it is a ritual practice based on the spiritual culture and established manners of the Japanese people. During the ceremony, the participants are required to smell, identify and then comment on the particular aroma and effect of 10 pieces of agar wood. The incense material used in the art of incense is limited to agar wood, which gives off various odours according to its age, the part used and the amount of resin it contains, etc. The art of incense is still practised in Japan, although it is not as well known as the tea ceremony, largely due to the lack of agar wood. Today, the aesthetic appreciation of incense is being revived, incense shops in Japan are offering new creations and incense study groups have sprung up. Apart from cultivating refinement of taste and discrimination, the incense ritual also helps train the mind and develop psychic concentration:

> If one can suspend any preconceptions about incense to fully experience the ceremony, the happy result will be the ability to appreciate 'incense time' as one would 'tea time' for relaxation, refreshment and communion with others.[7]

Like many other Far Eastern countries, the Japanese also favour sandalwood, which they still burn on their Shinto shrines (the pre-Buddhist religion of Japan). It is clear that the use of aromatics for ritual purposes in the Orient is still very much alive today, unlike the Western traditions, which reached a height during the Greek and Roman period before undergoing a gradual but widespread decline.

THE GREEKS AND ROMANS

The Greeks' love of aromatics and incense is deeply rooted in their history. Ritual incense burners or censers have been excavated from Minoan graves in Crete, dated to before 1500 BC. In *The Odyssey*, Homer (*c.* 850 BC) refers to an incense altar in the temple of Aphrodite at Paphos, in Cyprus. The goddess is supposed to have hidden her nakedness with a bough of myrtle and the fragrance of myrtle plays an important role in Greek incense ceremonies up to the present day.

In ancient times, the principal means by which the Greeks honoured their gods was by making human sacrifices and later by burning domestic animals. In the course of time, only a small portion of the meat was burned, together with libations (the pouring of wine) and incense, while the rest was consumed in a festive meal. By the sixth century BC, the Greek custom of making animal sacrifices had been largely replaced by the ritual offering of incense. A Greek inscription at Didyma (about 300 BC) lists frankincense, myrrh, cassia, cinnamon and costus being offered at the temple of Apollo.

The powdered type of incense was generally kept in a special box and burned either on an incense altar in the temple or at a household shrine using a brazier. At public festivals and military triumphs, censers containing incense were borne along by the procession, while large quantities were burned in front of temples and in niches and doorways along the processional route. At celebrations connected with the oracle at Delphi, Thessalian virgins carried baskets of incense and spices at the head of the procession.

Like the Egyptians, the Greeks also used incense to induce a change of consciousness. According to Plutarch, the Pythic Oracle at Delphi used a mixture of bay leaf and barley flour as an incense to help induce a trance-like state. Likewise, when the oracle at Patras was consulted, the priestess prayed and offered incense before gazing into the sacred well to seek an answer. It is more than likely that incense also played a prominent role in the 'miracle cures' of the priest-doctors of Asclepius – incenses are included in recipes on marble tablets within their temples.

At funerals, the Greeks burnt incense not only to propitiate the gods, but also as a symbol of transcendence. When cremation replaced burial rites, it also served the more practical purpose of disguising the odour of burning flesh and purifying the area of germs or infection.

It was the Romans, however, who began to use incense increasingly lavishly for this purpose, until vast sums were being squandered on it. It is reported that the whole of Arabia could not produce in a year as much incense as was burned in one day by the Emperor Nero upon the death of his consort, Poppaea. As Pliny pointed out laconically:

> Arabia's good fortune has been caused by the luxury of mankind even in the hours of death, when they burn over the departed the products which they had originally understood to have been created for the gods.[8]

With the Romans, incense also began to be used increasingly for secular rather than religious purposes. The Romans were renowned for their love of sweet-smelling perfumes and 'unguents', which they used to scent their hair, their bodies, their clothes, their beds, their baths and even the walls of their houses. Of frankincense, Ovid said, 'If it is pleasing to the Gods, it is no less useful to mortals'[9] and Plutarch observed that through scent alone, 'imaginary worries are smoothed like a mirror'.[10] Indeed, the enormous quantities of 'foreign essences' imported by the Romans, and the consequent pressure which incense and perfume put on the treasury, may have been a substantial factor in the final collapse of the Empire.

The Bible and the Jewish Tradition

Nowhere has the ritual use of incense been more exactly prescribed than in the Jewish tradition. When the Jews left Egypt in 1240 BC, they took many Egyptian customs with them, including their use of incense. During their exodus, Moses was given a number of commandments by the Lord, including instructions on how to construct an incense altar and make a holy incense:

> Take sweet spices: storax, onycha [labdanum], galbanum, sweet spices and pure frankincense in equal parts, and compound an incense, such a blend as the perfumer might make, salted, pure and holy. Crush a part of it into a fine powder, and put some of this in front of the Testimony in the Tent of Meeting, the place appointed for my meetings with you. You must

> regard it as most holy. You are not to make any incense of similar composition for your own use. You must hold it to be holy thing, reserved for Yahweh. Whoever copies it for use as a perfume shall be outlawed from his people.[11]

Incense, in this context, is regarded as something extremely precious and sacred – it is to be burned at the meeting-place of man and God. The high priests made their offerings in front of the curtains of the innermost sanctuary, but its use was forbidden to laymen. When Korah and his 250 followers rebelled against the priesthood, Moses and Aaron put them to the test by challenging them to carry censers filled with incense before the Tent of Meeting. Then the Lord appeared to the gathered crowd, destroyed the rebels with fire and ordered the bronze censers to be picked out of the ashes and hammered into sheets to cover the altar. Later, in order to protect the rest of the community, Moses said to Aaron:

> Take the censer, fill it with fire from the altar, put incense in it and hurry to the community to perform the rite of atonement over them. The wrath has come down from Yahweh and the plague has begun. Aaron did as Moses said and ran among the assembly, but the plague was already at work among them. He put in the incense and performed the rite of atonement over the people. Then he stood between the living and the dead, and the plague stopped.[12]

Here, incense is being used for purification purposes, not only to wash away the sins of the people, but also to kill infection and prevent disease from spreading, much in the same way as it was used during the Great Plague of 1665. The priestly habit of burning aromatics between themselves and the populace during a service also served as a protective barrier against germs. Likewise, the purification rites of Hebrew women employed many aromatics. In the year before marriage, it was customary for Hebrew women to undergo a purification ritual for six months using firstly oil of myrrh, followed by a further six months using frankincense and other scented unguents. Women also generally wore a small cloth bag containing myrrh and other aromatics suspended as a necklet between their breasts. The perfume was slowly released by contact with the body. It is clear from Mesopotamian and Biblical sources that women were particularly skilled in the art of perfumery and the employment of aromatic medicaments from early times.

After the Jews' arrival in 'The Promised Land', a guild of apothecaries or perfumers was set up. The most famous guild members belonged to the family of Abtinas. They acquired the monopoly of preparing the incense for temple worship and made about 370 lbs per annum (one mina for each day's offering plus three minas for the Day of Atonement). The incense was carried from the House of Abtinas by a chosen priest in a golden vessel. Then, while the congregation waited outside in silence, the priest threw the incense into the fire on the altar, bowed towards the Holy of Holies and carefully withdrew backwards. The rising incense smoke veiled the manifest form of Yahweh from the priest and congregation and protected them from the danger of his immediate holiness. Also, perhaps it was the pervasive fragrance of the burning incense itself that brought about the imminent presence of the deity.

Around the time of Christ, the Abtinas family asked the Temple aut horities for a price increase, which was turned down. When the Abtinas refused to divulge their formula, saying they feared that the incense might be used for idolatrous sacrifices, they were replaced by Egyptian apothecaries who had access to the original formula related to Moses – but who could not make the smoke ascend correctly. The Abtinas family were then reinstated at a substantially higher salary! According to Josephus, the Abtinas formula contained 13 ingredients, which, in addition to those listed in the original recipe, included myrrh, cassia, spikenard, saffron, costus, mace, cinnamon and their 'secret herb'. This last one imparted the property of making the smoke ascend in the shape of a date palm.

According to Maimonides, the Jewish physician and philosopher, the use of incense in the worship of the Jews actually originated from the practice of using aromatics to disguise the disagreeable odours arising from the burning of sacrificial animals, although he also mentions that it must have raised the spirits of the priests as well. Later, the scent of incense came to replace the odour of burnt offerings altogether. At this time the Hebrews believed, like the Egyptians, that the gods were nourished by odours and that all ethereal beings fed on vapours, not on solid food. On Mount Sinai, the Lord revealed to Moses how he would vent his fury if the people did not listen to him by smashing their incense altars so he could no longer breathe their appeasing fragrance

Incense, of course, was already in use throughout Israel at the time of the Jews' exodus from Egypt, and was in some areas an intrinsic part of their pagan form of worship. Excavations have revealed that there were at least seven different types of incense vessels in use during this period and that incense burning went back a far as chalcolithic times (fourth millennium BC) in Palestine. It is probable that the Israelites took over the Canaanite incense vessels which they used for the expression of local cult worship. It is clear that the priestly editors of the ancient traditions erased many elements of popular religion when they set about compiling the old Jewish texts, since they did not conform to their ideal.

Christianity and Modern Day Rituals

There can be little doubt that the scorn and revulsion with which incense was regarded in the early days of Christianity resulted from its heavy usage in pagan rituals and by the Jews. Consequently, for the first four centuries AD incense was used in Christian churches primarily as a sanitary aid rather than a religious tool. However, in the fourth century AD, Constantine the Great inaugurated the Peace of the Church which affirmed the use of incense in Christian practice in response to growing public pressure. Since then, some Christian sects have taken to using aromatics intensively as part of their ritual, while others have virtually abandoned its use altogether. The Coptic, Roman Catholic and Greek Orthodox Churches still use incense extensively, made mainly from frankincense, sometimes in combination with charcoal, benzoin and storax. During the Mass, the altar is incensed first as a symbol of the grace that suffused Christ like a sweet odour, then follows the incensing of the faithful, a reflection of the grace shed upon them by Christ.

In the West even today, however, the burning of incense in the form of joss-sticks, made mainly from east Indian and west Australian sandalwood, still carries the stigma of association with pagan worship to a certain extent.

In conclusion, it is clear that the ancients used incense extensively as part of their way of life. It was employed mainly in ritual practices for the following reasons:

1) as an offering or bloodless sacrifice – a symbol of wealth

2) as a way of uplifting and altering one's state of mind – to create the correct mood

3) as a means of 'communion' between the earthly and divine realm

4) as a protection against evil and to ensure favour

5) as a purifying agent for the psyche or soul of an individual

6) as a cleansing agent for physical body and the environment

7) as a pleasing perfume in meeting-places

But what is the basis for the universal employment of incense, in particular those ingredients derived from resins, woods and gums, as opposed to those from flowers, leaves or other sources? This was the question posed by the Syrian scholar Arnobius, in the fourth century AD. His scepticism undermines the whole concept underlying the ritual use of incense and could just as well be applied today:

> What is this sign of respect which comes from the smell of the gum of a tree burning in a fire? Does this, do you suppose, give honour to the heavenly magnates? Or if their displeasure has been aroused at any time, is it really soothed and dissipated by incense smoke? But if it is smoke the gods want, why do you not offer them any kind of smoke? Or must it only be incense? If you answer that incense has a nice smell while other substances have not, tell me if the gods have nostrils, and can smell with them? But if the gods are incorporeal, odours and perfumes can have no effect at all upon them, since corporeal substances cannot affect incorporeal beings.[13]

According to the psychologist Carl Jung, an important aspect in the development of individual consciousness may be understood as the process of withdrawing *projections*, *i.e.* the process of recognizing qualities previously ascribed to external factors as being potential aspects of oneself. Thus, the gods and goddesses of ancient mythologies or religions might in modern psychological language be seen as different *archetypes* or facets of the *Self*, rather than as separate external entities:

> All ages before ours believed in gods in some form or other. Only an unparalleled impoverishment in symbolism could enable us to discover the gods as psychic factors, which is to say, as archetypes of the unconscious. No doubt this discovery is hardly credible yet.[14]

Seen in this context, the use and effect of incense may be described in terms of its physiological and psychological impact on the human psyche.

In his book *The Scented Ape*, zoologist Michael Stoddard compares the scent of incense materials and their molecular composition with the make-up and odour of steroidal sex pheromones found in the human species. He concludes:

> Suffice it to say that the inspiration men get from incense is that it stimulates them in a truly profound manner, unconsciously stirring vestigial memory traces associated with times when odorous sex attractants played a vital role in the preservation of the species. There can be no odours more able to stimulate the deep emotional levels of the brain than those associated – however distantly and indistinctly – with sexual attraction.[15]

Viewed in this way, the scent of incense, reminiscent of sex attractant steroids, can help to lift conditioned repressive tendencies enough to release some of our deep-seated primitive emotions. Under the influence of incense, the rational mode of consciousness is diminished and the mind tends to become more alert and open to suggestion, and so it encourages a state where 'all minds think alike'. In 1977, Hines, a psychologist who has studied the effects of odours on the right cerebral hemisphere of the brain, firmly stated that:

> … odours are capable of inducing an ecstatic, emotional state of consciousness that would render individuals more susceptible to the sort of consciousness persuasion on which ritual and religious rites depend.[16]

Over the last decade a spate of research papers has been published on the psychological effects of odour and its potential uses. In addition, with the resurgence of interest in natural remedies and the growing concern for environmental issues which require a harmonious relationship with nature, the benefits of incense and aromatic materials are

Incense Table

The following botanical species are the most commonly used sources of incense:

Bark

borneol or Chinese camphor (Dryobalanops aromatica)

camphor (Cinnamomum camphora)

cassia (C. cassia)

cinnamon (C. zeylanicum)

Pollen

saffron (Crocus sativa)

Resins

balsam of Peru (Myroxylon pereirae)

balsam of tolu (M. toluiferum)

dragon's blood (Calamus draco)

elemi (Caanarium luzonicum)

frankincense (Boswellia sacra, B. carterii, etc)

galbanum (Ferula galbanifula)

ladanum (Cistus ladaniferus)

myrrh (Commiphora myrrha)

rose malloes (Liquidamber altungia)

styrax (Styrax officinalis, Liquidamber orientalis)

tragacanth (Astragalus gummifer)

Roots/Rhizomes

calamus (Acorus calamus)

costus (Auklandia costus)

spikenard (Nardostachys jatamansi)

Seed Coat

mace (Myristica fragrans)

Woods

aloes or eagle wood (Aquillaria agallochum)

cedar (Juniperus virginiana)

cypress (Cupressus torulosa)

juniper (Juniperus mexicana)

sandalwood (Santalum album)

---

being reassessed. The burning or vaporization of natural gums, resins and essential oils is already beginning to undergo a revival both at home and in society at large. Unlike synthetic air-fresheners, essential oils can be employed not only as anti-bacterial agents or to produce a pleasant smell, but also to reduce stress, aid relaxation, induce sleep, uplift and clear the mind or act as aphrodisiacs or euphorics. In their more traditional role, they can also help create a personal bridge to the sacred – through meditation, prayer, yoga, visualization or active imagination. As early as 1580, Montaigne, the prolific French writer, observed in his *Essay on Smells*:

> Physicians might … make greater use of scents than they do, for I have often noticed that they cause changes in me, and act on my spirits … which makes me agree with the theory that the introduction of incense and perfume into the churches … was for the purpose of raising our spirits, and of exciting and purifying our senses, the better to fit us for contemplation.[17]

The full potential of incense and aromatics in modern day rituals has yet to be fully explored!

References

1. Cited in Nielsen, K., *Incense in Ancient Israel,* E. J. Brill, 1986, p.9.
2. Le Guérer, A., *Scent: The Mysterious Power of Smell*, Chatto and Windus, 1993, p.120.
3. Nielsen, op. cit. p.10.
4. Ibid., p.28 (Assur level H-G, Tepe Gawra).
5. Ibid., p.25 (Tablet IX, Surpu Series).
6. From The Ritual Practice of the Riwo Sangcho (unpublished version).
7. Morita, K., *The Book of Incense*, Kodansha International, cited in *Aromatherapy Quarterly*, no.36, p.18.
8. Groom, N., *Frankincense and Myrrh*, Longman, 1981, p.14.
9. Tisserand, R., *The Art of Aromatherapy*, C. W. Daniel, 1985, p.28.
10. Sigismund, R., *Die Aromata*, C. F. Winterische Verlagshandlung, Leipzig, 1884, p.2.
11. Exodus 30: 37–7.
12. Numbers 17: 11–14.
13. Atchely, 1909, cited in Stoddart, D. M., *The Scented Ape*, Cambridge University Press, 1990, p.180.
14. Jung, C. G., *Collected Works*, vol. IX, p.72.
15. Stoddart, op. cit., p.203.
16. Ibid.
17. Ibid.

three 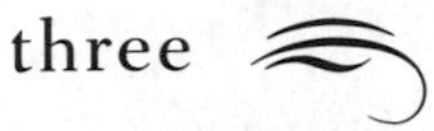

Scent, Soul and Psyche

The Wind One Brilliant Day …

The wind one brilliant day, called
to my soul with an aroma of jasmine.

'In return for this jasmine odor,
I'd like all the odor of your roses.'

'I have no roses; I have no flowers left now
in my garden … All are dead.'

'Then I'll take the waters of the fountains,
and the yellow leaves and dried up petals.'

The wind left … I wept. I said to my soul,
'What have you done with the garden entrusted to you?'

Antonio Machado, trans. Robert Bly, 1983.[1]

Why have we let the flowers die in the garden of our soul? Even the dried up petals have been blown away! Our present culture pays little attention to the needs of the heart – our emotional feeling nature has been subjugated to the constraints of reason for so long, that we now find ourselves in a spiritual wasteland. Compared to the great civilizations of the past, we do not honour enough the inner or unseen realm of the mind, the subtle expressions of the psyche. At one time, incense was burned upon temple altars and at household shrines on a daily basis, fragrant flowers were strewn on the floors of churches and dwelling-places, and the evocative power of perfume was understood as the silent language of divinity and human emotion. Now, having banished the ancient gods and goddesses, how are we to show our respect?

The Symbolic Imagination

> I do not feel like writing verses;
> but as I light my perfume-burner
> with myrrh, jasmine and incense,
> they suddenly burgeon from my heart,
> like flowers in a garden.[2]

Scent inspires the imagination and frees the spirit. In poetry, flowers are often used directly as a symbol of the soul, for their fragrance has an intangible quality which reaches out to our most intimate depths. To the primitive mind, the child's eye or the poet's pen, everything in the physical world can be seen as an expression of the more subtle, immaterial realm. To the ancients, there was far more to a plant than simply its tangible form, for each herb carried a whole series of associations with mythology, astrology and folklore. To the mind's eye, the scent, shape and colour of a plant, its habitat and manner of growth all helped to convey its innate quality. This essential, underlying property was known as the 'virtue'.

The bay tree, for example, with its radiant shining leaves, evergreen growth and narcotic, heady scent was associated with the sun, the sign of Leo, the god Apollo and the 'virtues' of strength, protection, courage, inspiration, prophecy and insight. The leaves were made into wreaths to crown victors and great artists or poets; it was planted by the door of houses to keep evil 'at bay'; and was used as incense by the *pythia*, the high priestess at the temple of Apollo in Delphi. When burned, herbs were seen to release their inner virtues. The scent of bay thus evoked the presence of Apollo, as well as the qualities of prophecy and clairvoyance needed by the *pythia* to transmit the message of the oracle.

John Gerard, in his popular herbal of 1597, esteemed scent before taste and before 'any confection of the apothecaries' for comforting the heart. In Britain, even up the Victorian age, the scent of a flower was believed to be its soul, and a fragrant bouquet was considered a time-honoured symbol of love and human passion. As romantic tokens, specific flowers were often used as metaphors for the range of the human emotions. A complex vocabulary was gradually developed, in which each flower was understood to represent a different mood or stage in the courtship procedure. In the language of flowers, the white lily stood for purity, innocence and virginity; the bluebell for loyalty, assurance and truth; and the mimosa for sensitivity and delicacy. A single red rose said 'I love you', but a bunch of mint meant 'Find a spouse of your own age and background'! The names of some flowers spoke for themselves, such as forget-me-not, heartsease or love-lies-bleeding.

Many flowers and plants have retained a ritual significance, though the original meaning has been lost. Kissing beneath a sprig of mistletoe at Christmas harks back to an old pagan custom when it was hung in the house throughout the year as a symbol of peace, friendship and goodwill.

The Chinese especially have always endowed certain plants and flowers with symbolic attributes, for example, the aged and crooked pine tree stands for virtue triumphant in adversity. The much loved and fragrant cassia was admired by poets chiefly for its perfume and, according to myth, grew on the moon – possibly because its scent was strongest at night! In the Chinese tale *Dream of the Red Chamber*, the noble family's impending collapse is presaged in the garden by a begonia which suddenly bursts into flower in mid-November. Reversals of nature cannot but bode ill, for they reflect an inner lack of harmony which sooner or later leads to disaster. On the other hand, the vigorous but unexceptional blossoming of common plants such as the orchid or chrysanthemum signify that all is well within the household.

In Western fairy tales, trees and plants are often involved as life tokens, the life force of a person being involved with a tree planted at birth. In the Grimms' story *The Juniper Tree*, a murdered boy is buried beneath a juniper tree with his mother, only to be reborn like a phoenix from its depths:

> Then the juniper tree began to stir itself, and the branches parted asunder, and moved together again, just as if someone were rejoicing and clapping his hands. At the same time a mist seemed to arise from the tree, and in the centre of this mist it burned like a fire, and a beautiful bird flew out of the fire, singing magnificently, and he flew high up in the air, and when he was gone, the juniper tree was just as it had been before.[3]

In this story, the juniper tree is the source of new life and hope from which the released soul arises. In the original myth of the phoenix, the fire-bird dies and is reborn from the aromatic ashes of fragrant wood. The 'spiritual bird' arises from the depths of the pyre like incense from a fragrant fire. Indeed, the ancient Egyptians believed that the phoenix first brought incense to the Land of Punt in his claws and that the scent of incense was his own scent. The Hebrews thought the phoenix was a god reincarnated and the Egyptians saw him as the soul of Osiris, the god whose breath smelt of myrrh and incense. According to the Egyptian legend, at the end of his long life, the phoenix builds himself a nest of frankincense and cassia on which he dies, and from his corpse arises the new phoenix. Thus the phoenix, like scent, depicts the vital essence or spark of life, the immortal soul; in this sense it can be equated with the 'fire-water' of the shamans and with the 'quintessence' of the alchemists. As Gaston Bachelard says in *Fragments d'une poetique du feu*, 'Odours in and of themselves make myths possible ...'

Slowly, however, with the growth of rationalism in the West, the symbolic imagination was repressed – only poets and children were allowed to speak in the language of the heart:

> Rational thought, in its pursuit of objective knowledge, denies the validity of subjective visualisation. Its diabolic methodology has supplanted the symbolic perspective, and the material world is perceived as existing in its own right quite dissociated from the person observing it.[4]

Yet the symbolism that has accumulated around particular plants or flowers in the course of time, together with the significance of their fragrance, is still very much a part of our collective cultural conditioning today. This underlying mythic language still communicates itself, often via the unconscious, and conditions our response both to its form and to its scent. Symbolism and myth still speak to us in the language of the unseen, just as scent communicates itself to our soul directly, influencing our mood and emotions in a subtle manner.

The gods and goddesses are not dead – it is just that we no longer see them or believe in them! To reawaken their power is to reinvest matter with spirit, to perceive the virtues concealed within the external manifestation of form. The virtues of the deities reside within ourselves and in nature; the virtues of plants express themselves through scent and through their 'essence'. To honour the presence of the spirit within is to become attuned to a way of seeing using the 'mind's eye' and the symbolic imagination.

The Odour of Sanctity

Certain flowers have always tended to attract a spiritual significance or symbolism, just as certain scents have always been associated with an experience of the sacred, notably the rose. The Persian writer, Avicenna, dedicated a whole book to the spiritual and medicinal virtues of his favoured plant, the rose. Among the Sufis, the experience of the divine is intimately associated with the form and scent of the Queen of Flowers:

> And above all, the repeated splendours of glowing dawns, the profusion of rose gardens, white roses and red roses, the shades of the rose bushes, the divine presence flashing in the brilliance of a red rose.[5]

The rose and its fragrance have been associated with love and feminine beauty in all cultures alike from time immemorial. Dedicated to Venus/Aphrodite, the very scent has a sensual and rich allure. Yet the rose is also associated with the heart and has always been used symbolically to indicate religious passion or devotion. The Madonna is often depicted in a garden of roses in icon paintings. Here, the rose indicates Mary's love for the child Jesus, while more profoundly it suggests the love required for the nurturing of the Christ principle within. According to tradition, the Virgin appeared to St Dominic bearing a chaplet of roses, and the first rosary of beads (made from compressed rose leaves) was made in commemoration of this vision. In the esoteric Western tradition, the appearance of angels is also said to be accompanied by the aroma of roses!

Celestial scents have often accompanied religious experiences. Charles Fourier's vision of souls in heaven took the form of 'aromatic bodies' floating about within an 'aromatic shell' which surrounded the planet like a bubble, while in the Islamic esoteric text *The Jasmine of the Fedeli d'amore*, Rûzbehân experienced the celestial world as being suffused with wondrous perfumes:

> The love of ardent desire was born in my heart and I felt my heart merge with that love. I spent all the time in deep nostalgia, for then my heart plunged into the Ocean of Memory of eternal pre-existence and into the scent of the perfumes of the celestial world.[6]

Later he describes a vision of a ritual of inner ascent in which he saw himself as if from above, being initiated into another realm of understanding. The substance which is used to mark the transition is aromatics:

> He notices that a pot is suspended, under which there burns a pure and smokeless subtle fire, fed by odoriferous herbs . . . The Shayk breaks one of the loaves into the bowl and pours the contents of the pot into it. 'It was,' our mystic says, 'a kind of oil, but something very subtle, of a totally spiritual nature.'[7]

In many cultures, there are also documented experiences of the 'odour of sanctity' – a certain undefinable smell which surrounds holy men or women. According to first-hand accounts of this phenomenon, there is not simply an odour of sanctity, but a whole range of sacred scents. The record of Hubert Larcher describes St Lyddwyne de Schiedam's odour as having seven components: cinnamon, cut flowers, ginger, clove, lily, rose and violet. St Teresa of Avila's scent, on the other hand, consisted of lily and orris, and changed after her death to include violet and jasmine. Like secular perfumes, holy odours changed and ripened with the course of time, and could even last long after the physical body was dead. A witness who examined St Teresa's body 12 years after her demise remarked upon 'the sweet odour it released, the freshness and beauty of the seemingly still living flesh'.[8]

In historical or mythic terms, the odour of sanctity probably originated in ancient Egypt, where the souls of the dead were judged by Anubis, the jackal-headed Lord of the Underworld. With his keen nose he was able to smell the 'essence' of each person and thus determine the purity of their soul. In this sense, a person's odour reflects their inner depth, their soul quality.

Those seeking a more rational explanation for the cause of the 'odour of sanctity' have come up with a variety of theories based mainly on somatic or pathological changes in the blood. Dr Hubert Larcher, however, has advanced a view suggesting that mystical life could result in a dramatic slowing down of the metabolism and that ecstatic states may result in the formation of 'odoriferous compounds' within the organism:

> Ultimately the condition of the soul controls a chemistry capable of removing some of its somatic links and thus of helping it to take wing.[9]

He further suggests that the alcohols pumped into the blood during the ecstatic state could lead to a kind of mystical intoxication, which, like certain drugs, could open the 'doors of perception' and induce visionary experiences. The shared 'celestial visions' reported by the nuns who surrounded St Teresa's deathbed may be related to this process, bearing in mind 'the possible action of the molecules involved in the odour of sanctity – which was especially strong and almost unbearable – on the nervous system and psychic functioning of those nuns'.[10]

The Doors of Perception

Using aromatics and herbal drugs to open the doors of perception was a domain of expertise specific to the traditional shaman. The shaman featured largely in primitive forms of medicine because he or she was able to travel back and forth across the invisible barrier that divides matter from spirit, and act as a mediating influence:

> The shaman himself must be a master of psychological control ... he rejoins that which was once a totality – man and the animals, the living and the dead, man and the gods ... and in providing this integration, the shaman provides his magical cure.[11]

Within a contemporary context, the shaman's magical flight could be seen as a form of psycho-therapeutic practice. Indeed, the key to health from the shamanic perspective was seen to lie predominantly in the domain of the psyche – and one of the principal ways of gaining access to this realm was by the use of herbs and aromatics.

An important part of the shaman's rigorous and challenging training was acquiring knowledge about medicinal plants, including those with hallucinogenic powers. Those plants which had curious psychic effects included aromatics such as hemlock (*Conium maculatum*), mugwort

(*Artimesia vulgaris*), bay (*Lauris nobilis*), nutmeg (*Myristica fragrans*) and cannabis (*Cannabis sativa*).

Such knowledge has survived to the present day. In 1985, the Chumash medicine woman Chequeesh told researcher Will Noffke that she had learned of her native heritage by utilizing the 'dream herb' mugwort – a plant which is used to produce a narcotic (and toxic) essential oil. Hem-lock, a poisonous aromatic plant with a foetid smell, was a vital part of the European witch's arsenal, and enabled her to fly away on her broomstick – the equivalent of the shaman's magical flight. In the Hindu Kush, the sibyl inhales fragrant smoke from the sacred cedar in order to induce a trance-like state before pronouncing the oracle, much in the same way as the *pythia* of Delphi. On the island of Madura, off the north coast of Java, the spirit medium, generally a woman, sits with her head over a censer of incense for some time, until she is overcome and eventually collapses. Upon recovery, her voice is purportedly that of the spirit which has taken over her soul. In Uganda, the mediums first have to light up a herbal pipe and repeatedly inhale deeply until they have worked themselves up to a frenzy, at which point the gods speak through them.

In eastern Asia and the Orient, shamanism and animism predate the more familiar mainstream religions like Buddhism, Confucianism and Hinduism. Cannabis was being used in India and China as early as 1500 BC for sacred ceremonial purposes, and the ancient Scythians used it in the form of a narcotic vapour bath. The main active constituents in cannabis are a resin and a volatile oil: the Indian name for this part of the herb is *charas*. It is the resinous exudation from the aerial parts which contains a large percentage of a red essential oil. In India today it is still smoked by the *sadus* or wandering holy men as part of their religious life. Since cannabis or marijuana is also commonly used in the West as a mind-altering drug, there can be no doubt that certain aromatics can have a profound effect on the psyche or consciousness of an individual.

However, many of the so-called 'magical' herbs or oils are dangerous if they are not handled correctly and used in the right proportion. Such substances can easily be misused and abused if their power is not respected. As the Native American medicine man Chief Maza Blaska of the Ogallalla tribe says:

> From Wakan-Tanka, the Great Mystery, comes all power. It is from Wakan-Tanka that the Holy Man has wisdom and the power to heal and to make holy charms. Man knows that all healing plants are given by Wakan-Tanka; therefore are they holy.[12]

Implicit in the ancient use of herbs and aromatics for healing purposes was an awareness of the sacred dimension within the ritual and the need for a correct attitude to the process for it to be effective. The fragrant plants which were used to make holy oils or incense for fumigation were often seen as having an identity in their own right, a personality which had to be respected if they were to work. Healing rituals were often accompanied by chants or incantations which honoured the soul or spirit of the plant. In ancient Egypt, hymns were sung to Nefertum, 'god of the sacred lotus', a plant renowned for its narcotic properties:

> I invoke Nefertum, in the following of Ptah. Thou art guardian and protector of the perfume and oil makers, protector and god of the sacred lotus. Osiris is the body of the plants, Nefertum is the soul of the plants, the plants purified. The divine perfume belongs to Nefertum living forever.[13]

The scent of the lotus was identified with the soul, its immortal aspect. It is also known that the ancient Egyptians pressed the lotus blossoms to acquire their juice. Added to wine, this 'perfumed extract' would produce a powerful psychoactive drug, which could produce visionary experiences or dreams. The fragrance scholar Morris noted that this is the 'first instance of the association of inhalation of perfumes with inhalation of hallucinogens'.[14] Medicinal plants and aromatics were thus used to open the doors of perception or gain access to the realm of the unseen, so as to restore unity. The importance of the spiritual dimension on such a journey was vital for the success of the healing operation, as well as for the personal safety of the shaman/priest, acting on behalf of the troubled soul.

THE SUBTLE ESSENCE

> The essence is like the personality or spirit of the plant. It is the most ethereal and subtle part of the plant and its therapeutic action takes place on a higher and more subtle level, having in general a much more pronounced effect on the mind and emotions.[15]

Shamanic practices are still in evidence in various parts of the world. In South America, for example, certain shamans called *perfumeros* actually perform their cure specifically through fragrances. They are especially sensitive to the nuances of body odour, and seek to transform the 'aura' of their patient by manipulating their diet and prescribing plant aromas.

> Both the rainforest Indians and the Mestizos, the mixed Spanish–Indian population use perfumes, floral waters and aromatic plants in their healing rituals ... The basic idea is that good smelling fragrances protect against bad spirits by strengthening the aura, whereas bad smelling fragrances, like rotting meat, damage the aura. The aura is considered to be the energetic-emotional envelope around the body. Each tribe has a classification of good and bad smells.[16]

As part of the ritual, the shaman often takes *ayahuasca*, a hallucinogenic jungle vine, which enables him or her to discern or smell the cause of the illness, which is usually attributed to evil spirits or sorcery. Tobacco is also revered as a magical plant throughout the Amazon and used to communicate with and nourish the spirit world. Some tribes use the scent of the Amazonian basil (*Ocimum mircanthum*) to relieve anxiety and banish fearful visions. The Kuripakos of the Amazon collect the solidified resin from the *Protium crassipetalium* and burn it to 'purify the house' following an illness.

> The Mestizos say that shamans cannot do a proper healing without perfume. They have an altar of Christian and native power objects which must be purified and activated before a curing ceremony can take place. They say that fragrance is the link that holds all of these power objects together for healing, so it is essential.[17]

Often while in a trance state, the shaman hears and sings magical healing songs while using a bunch of herbs to beat out a rhythm. The healing is also carried out in various other ways – sometimes the patient is given an aromatic bath and then rubbed with fragrant oils; sometimes the shaman puts some perfume into his or her own mouth, and after inhaling tobacco smoke, sprays it on to the patient. This is called *florecer*, which means 'to blossom' or to make whole. The shaman's breath is also thought to have a healing power and the breath itself is considered a vehicle for the revitalization of the soul.

> Just as the soul, or essence, of mankind had to be persuaded to depart temporarily through fumigation in order for a spirit to enter the oracle, so it was commonly thought among many peoples that the soul would leave the body with the last breath at death . . . The common themes running through these observations are the notions that the breath, the soul and odour are in some way interconnected, and that a being can be protected from evil outside influences in much the same way as the gods can be assuaged.[18]

In *Perfume: The Story of a Murderer*, Süskind also identifies essence with breath, and breath as the medium which carries scent, unlike words, pictures or sounds, into the very soul of a person:

> For scent was a brother to breath. Together with breath it entered human beings, who could not defend themselves against it, not if they wanted to live. And scent entered into their very core, went directly to their hearts, and decided for good and all between affection and contempt, disgust and lust, love and hate. He who ruled scent ruled the hearts of men.[19]

In this context, it is interesting to note that the olfactory cells are also the only place in the human body where the central nervous system is directly in contact with the external environment. When we smell something, there is a direct contact between the molecules of the scent and our own receptors – it is an intimate or *essential* type of encounter. While neurones of the visual or auditory system lead to the brain's *cortex*, the seat of abstract reasoning and analysis, the neurones of the olfactory system lead to the *hypothalamus*, which controls the subjective experience or 'inner' response – memories, feelings, moods and the body's hormones.

Vibrational Healing

A contemporary healer who, like the traditional shaman, has access to the spirit or supernatural world, has been told that he had been given a *dimensional doorway* which made him open to a vast store of energy. During his healing sessions, he manifests aromatic oils and ash, which literally pour from his hands, filling the room with scent.

> ...the interesting thing is that the aromatic oil will often start as one aroma and when a person has received it, their energy takes over and it might change several times. It's personalised to them...[20]

The idea that aromas can be 'personalized' to an individual corresponds with Marguerite Maury's method of revitalizing her patients using a 'strictly personal aromatic complex' or 'individual prescription' which was perfectly adapted to that person's temperament and state of health. Present-day writing on astral magic also emphasizes the value of specific personalized perfumes as a medium for healing. According to one theory, odours created by the volatilization of particles of matter emit vibrations that have a profound effect on the behaviour of all living creatures and especially on their 'astral double' or 'aura':

> A perfume adapted to a person's astral sign will therefore tend to maintain his native humoral balance and auto-immune reactions through the unconscious reactions it provokes in the organism. It thereby acts as a charm that will enable the individual to improve his natural abilities and avoid imbalances. Each sign of the zodiac and each day of the month correspond to specific propitious aromas.[21]

Some ancient writers even allotted a perfume to each day of the week: saffron on Sunday; mastic on Monday; cassia on Tuesday; cinnamon on Wednesday; aloes on Thursday; ambergris on Friday; musk on Saturday. By association, the fragrances are used to evoke or to form a link with the archetypal forces they represent. The choice of scent should therefore be attuned to the needs and personality of the individual if it is to be effective (see also Chapter 6). In *Magical Aromatherapy*, Scott Cunningham explores the 'merging of human and plant energy' and the way essential oils or *ethereal oils* (as they are called in Germany) can be utilized together with visualization to manifest specific changes.

Like traditional shamans, contemporary spiritual healers see essential oils as having a particular affinity with the subtle energy or 'aura' of an individual, and having a revitalizing and harmonizing effect. In *Subtle Aromatherapy*, Patricia Davis further investigates the connection of essential oils with the chakras of the body, and the way in which they can be used to activate and balance energy within the subtle body. The base chakra for example, is associated with patchouli, myrrh, vetiver, frankincense and elemi; the heart with rose, inula, bergamot, melissa and jasmine. In the practice of subtle aromatherapy it is 'the vibration or subtle energy of the plant which is the healing factor'. This is, however, harder to explain or examine than the physical properties of medicinal plants. Davis continues:

> ...so how can we set about discovering these subtle healing properties? We can take a look at how plants have been used in the past, in shamanic traditions, in the ceremonial of many different religions, their symbolism in art, their meaning in myth and folklore ... Finally we can study the plants themselves, for they can tell us much about their hidden abilities.[22]

Examining the traditions of the past with an open yet discriminating eye is a key to the future understanding of plant medicine, including the psychological effects of aromatic oils. Another great tradition which spanned the centuries, burying its roots deep into the underlying cultural ethos of both East and West, and concerning itself with the investigation of essential oils and the soul, was that of alchemy.

The Quintessence of the Alchemists

> Alchemists at one time used a process by which they produced metal out of herbs, and another process by which they extracted the essence of flowers in such a way that one drop of it spread its perfume for miles. That art seems to have been lost; yet what we can learn from it is that in everything that exists there is a spirit, and that spirit has all the qualities which the outside of that thing shows least.[23]

At the heart of the alchemical operation was the quest for the *prima materia*, or the Philosopher's Stone. Called by a multitude of names, this mysterious substance was said to have an imperfect body, a constant soul, a penetrating tincture and a clear transparent mercury, volatile and mobile. The whole of the 'Work' was to be prepared and achieved with this single substance, which the alchemists believed to be the 'quintessence' of life itself. In order to produce this mysterious 'elixir' and turn the 'gross' into the 'subtle', the alchemist had to follow a complicated procedure known as *solve et coagula* – dissolve and combine. This process of refinement, which was carried out using a distillation vessel, included four stages – separation, extraction, fusion and sublimation – which were performed over and over again. We know today that the alchemists' pursuit of elemental transmutation was on the wrong track, but what they did discover was a profound parallel between the material and immaterial world, between natural and spiritual laws. On the material plane, the alchemist was concerned with discovering the primary element of creation, the quintessence, which could transmute base metals into gold and confer longevity. On a psychological level, the alchemical task involved the transformation of the human psyche and the perfecting of the soul.

Alchemy thus represented both a physical and a psychological process, where both levels were concerned with *essence*. But whereas the tradition of conscious, inner alchemy descended mainly from the Islamic, Greek and Oriental philosophies, the type of alchemy which aimed at rejuvenating or preserving the physical body was derived from Egyptian practice. The Egyptians were experts in the medicinal and cosmetic effects of essential oils on the human body and utilized them in the mummification process. Stacte (oil of myrrh) was rubbed into the whole body and used to pack the inside of the corpse once the viscera had been removed. Styrax, nard and other spices and resins were also used. The Egyptians believed that the gods exuded a sweet odour and a safe passage to the after-life could only be assured if the body smelt sweet. Since there was an association between sweet odours and sanctity, it was not suprising that the priests, wishing to emulate Osiris, chewed cedar gum to perfume their breath. A late papyrus reads:

> The perfume of Arabia has been brought to thee, to make perfect thy smell through the scent of the God. Here are brought to thee liquids which are come from Ra, to make perfect thy smell in the Hall of Judgement. O sweet-smelling soul of the great God, thou dost contain such a sweet odour that thy face shall neither change nor perish. Thy

> members shall become young in Arabia and thy soul shall appear over thy body in Taneter.[24]

After this incantation the priest anointed the body with 10 sacred perfumes – their passport to the after-life. In attempting to secure immortality, the alchemists naturally looked to specific aromatics in their search for the 'elixir of life'. In Egyptian alchemy, one such substance, known as *didi*, was a narcotic drug made from lotus-laced wine. Taken as a medicine, this magical substance was thought to confer longevity or even immortality.

In Chinese alchemy, the quest for the elixir of life is illustrated by the story of Chao Ch'u of Shang-tang who was left for dead in a cave in the mountains. There a genie found him and gave him a pouch of medicine which enabled him to live for over 300 years, without ever suffering the ill-health of old age. When asked for the contents of the pouch, the genie replied, 'This is only pine resin, very abundant on this mountain. Just refine this substance and take it, and you will enjoy Fullness of Life and Immortality.'[25]

But the ancient alchemists were well aware of the potential curative effects of essential oils and aromatics on the mind as well as on the body. With regard to the mind, Theophrastus Paracelsus wrote about the power of aromatics as substances which could 'take away diseases from patients just as civet destroys ordure, with its odour'.[26] Just as good odours cancelled out bad odours, aromatic oils counteracted infection and illness, and were especially beneficial in cases of mental disturbances:

> By means of the odoriferous specifics diseases are cured in persons who cannot take medicines, as in cases of apoplexy and of epilepsy. Many odours exist which relieve the epileptic; and many too which aid the apoplectic. They may not cure them, but they pave the way for a cure …[27]

It is interesting to note that the fragrance of various essential oils, especially ylang ylang, is currently being used in the treatment of epilepsy, with considerable success.

The Perfecting of the Soul

By the end of the Middle Ages, the Work of alchemy had begun to develop into a concise *mystical system*. Then in the fifteenth and sixteenth centuries, the experiences of generations of alchemists were 'distilled' into a unified doctrine: the *opus alchymicum*. Seen in this context, the whole process of distillation could be seen as a metaphor for human spiritual development or the 'perfecting of the soul' through the dynamic interaction of Matter and Spirit.

At the beginning, Matter and Spirit are infused together in a 'gross' manner – this is the *prima materia*. Then, through the application of heat (the fire of the instincts), Spirit begins to separate from Matter, much as the distillate rises to the top of the alembic vessel leaving the gross material behind. This stage requires the sacrifice of old notions or outworn patterns of behaviour, so the spirit – the pure innate quality of human nature – can arise. At the next stage, Matter attracts Spirit back to it, just as the volatile distillate recondenses to form a liquid, rather than remaining in an airy state. Finally, Matter and Spirit are reunited in a transformed state, the *mystic marriage*or *conjunctio* of the alchemists. This marriage reflects the conscious union of the human soul with the godhead, symbolized by the quintessence. In old alchemical texts, this resulting quintessence or essential oil was often called the 'volatile sulphur' and was also known as the 'soul' or the 'Apollo'.

Volatile oils, by their very nature, symbolize the soul, being an emanation of matter – manifestation of spirit. An old alchemical name for the soul was *aqua oleum*, meaning 'water-oil'. Essential oils partly resemble water and partly oil: they partake of both qualities yet they have their own nature. Water and oil don't mix – in fact they are as diametrically opposed as mind and matter. Like essential oils, the soul partakes of both the material and spiritual aspects, yet retains its own immutable quality. Like the soul, essential oils bridge the gap between the spirit/mind and the instincts/body, and in this context they are alchemical mediators or 'messengers of the soul', able to influence and touch both the mind and body.

> Essential oils ... could be seen as a bridge forming an almost intangible link between the 'two worlds' of spirit and matter ... we have not only the material aspect of the oil ... but also the ethereal aroma which influences the spiritual aspect.[28]

In his interpretation of the Grimms' fairy tale *Spirit in a Bottle*, Jung shows that in simple terms this story contains the quintessence or deepest meaning of the Hermetic mystery, which is at the heart of alchemy as it has come down to us today. In the story, a young boy finds a spirit called Mercurius trapped in a bottle at the foot of an oak tree. When the boy opens the bottle the spirit threatens to strangle him, but the young lad is able to trick it back into confinement. Then, in exchange for his freedom, the spirit offers the boy the reward of wealth together with the power of healing. The boy accepts.

> The mention of Mercurius stamps the fairy tale as an alchemical folk legend, closely related on the one hand to the allegorical tales used in teaching alchemy and on the other to the well-known group of fairy tales that cluster round the motif of the 'spellbound spirit'. Our fairy tale thus interprets the evil spirit as a pagan god, forced under the influence of Christianity to descend into the dark underworld and be morally disqualified ... In fact the spirit in the bottle behaves just as the devil does in many other fairy tales: he bestows wealth by changing base metal into gold; and like the devil, he also gets tricked.[29]

This fairy story presents in many ways an allegory of the evolution of the human soul or consciousness, as represented by the 'spirit/genie' in the bottle. In its rejection of nature, the West denied the possibility of an individual relationship to divinity and, by extension, the very existence of the soul, by burying it deep underground. Yet the soul was itself always contained deep in the psyche (at the foot of the oak tree), only to re-emerge transformed at a later date, bringing with it the 'gifts' of wealth and healing. In alchemical terms, Matter is attracting Spirit back to it: the vapour is recondensing!

This emerging 'totality' figure, which Jung calls the 'Self', represents a new orientation in consciousness which corresponds to what in religious language could be termed a submission of 'my will' to 'Thy will'. However, within the psychological framework of alchemy, the experience of the divine is seen as emerging from within, as opposed to via the religious experience of an external Godhead.

References

1. Reprinted from *Times Alone: Selected Poems of Antonio Machado*, Wesleyan University Press, 1993, with kind permission of Robert Bly.
2. Hafiz, fourteenth century.
3. Grimm Brothers, *The Complete Grimms' Fairytales*, Routledge and Kegan Paul, 1975, p.224.
4. Warren-Davis, D., 'Reading Between the Lines' in *International Federation of Aromatherapists*, Autumn 1990, p.9.
5. Corbin, H., 'The Jasmine of the Fedeli D'Amore' in Cobb, N., and Loewe, E., *Sphinx 3, A Journal for Archetypal Psychology and the Arts*, Claughton Press, 1990, p.201.
6. Ibid., p.195.
7. Ibid., p.200.
8. Bollandistus, *Acta Sanctorum* (1643), cited in Larcher, H., *Le sang, peut-il vaincre la mort?*, Paris Gallimard, 1957, p.27.
9. Ibid., p.221.
10. Ibid., p.222.
11. Myerhoff, B., *American Folk Medicine*, University of California Press, 1976, p.100.
12. Cited in Thomson, W. A. R., *Healing Plants – A Modern Herbal*, Macmillan, 1978, p.8.
13. Eighteenth Dynasty (1550–1295 BC), Cairo; Steele, J., 'The Transformational Use of Fragrance in Ancient Egypt and South American Shamanism' in Dodd, G. H. and Van Toller, S., *Fragrance: The Psychology and Biology of Perfume II*, Elsevier Science Publications Ltd., 1992, p.290.
14. Cited ibid., p.291.
15. Comito, T., *The Idea of the Garden in the Renaissance*, Harvester Press, 1979, p.32.
16. Steele, J., 'In Profile' in *The International Journal of Aromatherapy*, vol.5, no.1, 1993, p.8.
17. Ibid.
18. Stoddart, D. M., *The Scented Ape*, Cambridge University Press, 1990, p.123.
19. Süskind, P., *Perfume: The Story of a Murderer*, Hamish Hamilton, London, 1986, p.86.
20. Boltwood, G., 'Hands That Heal' in *Kindred Spirit*, vol.2, no.7, p.22.
21. LeGuèrer, A., *Scent: The Mysterious Power of Smell*, Chatto and Windus, 1993, p.6.
22. Davis, P., *Subtle Aromatherapy*, C. W. Daniel, 1991, p.52.
23. Hazrat Inayat Khan, *Philosophy, Psychology and Mysticism*, vol.XI.
24. Atchley, 1909, cited in Stoddart, op. cit., p.169.
25. Ware, J. R., trans., *Alchemy, Medicine and Religion in the China of AD 320*, The M.I.T. Press, 1966, p.193.

26. Paracelsus, T., 'Concerning the Odoriferous Specific' in Waite, A. E., *The Hermetic and Alchemical Writings of Paracelsus*, vol.II, T. Elliott & Co., Berkeley, 1976, p.61.
27. Ibid.
28. Wildwood, C., *Creative Aromatherapy*, Thorsons, 1993, p.18.
29. Jung, C. G., 'Alchemical Studies' (1944) in *The Collected Works*, vol.13, Routledge and Kegan Paul, 1959, p.198.

four 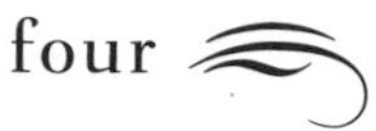

The Allure of Perfume

Fragrance of the orange
Flowering at last in June
Wafts through the Summer night
The memory of scented sleeves
Of someone long ago.

Kokinshu III: 139, Anon.

Perfumes have been used by humankind since the beginning of recorded history. Mention is made in ancient Chinese texts of materials used for perfumery over 8,000 years ago. In China, the legendary Yellow Emperor is attributed with bringing the first medicines and perfumes to the world, while in India the birth of perfumery is attributed to the god Indra. In Japan, it was common at all times for both sexes to carry a little box called *Inro* attached to their kimono sash, containing herbal remedies and fragrant love potions. Aromatics were, and still are, an intrinsic part of life in the Far East.

The Orientals were probably the first people to become familiar with the art of perfumery and the power of fragrance. In the Indus Valley, at the foot of the Himalayas, delicate perfume containers and perfectly preserved terracotta distillation equipment used for the extraction of essential oils point to the existence of a civilization with a sophisticated knowledge and utilization of aromatics some 5,000 years ago.

The East has always had many highly scented gums, resins and oils at its disposal, but little is known about the exact recipes and rituals of this ancient period. It is to the Egyptians and the Greeks that one must look for the earliest documents describing the precise preparation of perfumes and specific directions for their use.

The Divine Origin of Perfume

> Perfumes, sacrifices and unctions exist and spread their odours everywhere, they open the portals of the elements and the heavens whereby man can glimpse through them the secrets of the creator.[1]

The divine origin of perfume is clear from the ancient Egyptian term for perfume: 'fragrance of the gods'. Special priests were in charge of the preparation of perfumes, which were made in small chambers or 'laboratories' within the temple precincts. The recipes for the various remedies and perfumes were said to have been originally transmitted by the god Thoth, so when the priests prepared the scents they had to do it in strict accordance with holy texts.

The Egyptians, like other ancient people, had no scents dissolved in alcohol, but only perfumed greases – solid or liquid fats charged with odour, called unguents. Since animal fats and vegetable oils absorbed odours, one of the most important methods of extracting fragrance was by using an early form of enfleurage, where the oil or fat was allowed to become saturated with scent from aromatic materials. Some herbal extracts were also prepared by means of maceration or infusion in water, while others were produced by simple expression or pressure. According to Dioscorides, the Egyptians also used a primitive form of distillation to produce essential oils. He describes a process in which cedar resin was slowly heated in a vessel, over which was suspended a bundle of wool. As the essential oil evaporated, the vapour collected and condensed in the wool, which was then squeezed out.

Essential oils, vegetable oils, fats, resins and gums were thus combined to make viscous perfumes, which were sometimes made solid enough to be formed into cones or balls. A papyrus dated 1500 BC shows cones of unguent being fixed onto the heads of Egyptian men and women in preparation for a ceremonial occasion. These were designed to gradually melt in the course of the evening, scenting their hair, their skin and the air around them. The Egyptians had over 30 different aromatic preparations and seven principal perfumes. At this time there was no clear distinction between perfumes, incense and herbal remedies, all of which were compounded from natural organic materials. Indeed, as we have seen, 'perfume' is derived from the Latin *per fumen* meaning 'to smoke', thereby indicating its original association with incense and fumigation. Thus aromatics played an essential role in most ritual practices, which tended to combine religious, therapeutic and social elements.

That perfumes were in great evidence in ancient Egypt is demonstrated by the vast amounts of perfume containers which have been discovered in the tombs. These were usually made of stone or alabaster with tight-fitting lids to keep the contents cool and were often beautifully fashioned. Delicate jars carved in alabaster which once contained perfumed oils are now exhibited in the British Museum and have been dated to about 3500 BC. Similar finely wrought stone jars have also been found in the ancient Minoan remains on Crete. The later Greeks and Romans tended to use decorated pottery containers or special vases made from Athenian ceramic called *aryballos* for their aromatic oils. It was only after the first century BC that glass perfume bottles began to be used.

In the Minoan palace at Zakros in eastern Crete, destroyed in about 1500 BC, a perfumers' workshop has been plausibly identified, containing braziers on perforated stands, incense burners, perfume jars and specialized equipment for the preparation of essential oils.[2] The Mycenaeans at Pylos had developed a highly organized industry in perfumed oil by the late thirteenth century BC, thereby giving perfume great economic value as well as important ritual significance. Perfumed oil was offered to the gods as grave gifts and small stirrup jars which were used to contain the oil abound in Mycenaean tombs all over mainland Greece.

The perfumed oil was also offered to the Mycenaean gods and used to anoint the deities' statues, a practice common all over the ancient world, especially in Egypt and the Near East. The Egyptians anointed their mummies and gods with an oil and water emulsion. Stacte or oil of myrrh was considered to be the supreme fragrance or 'ambrosia' of the gods. Likewise, the Hindus washed their idols with musk, sandal and other fragrant woods on a daily basis, while the Buddhist liturgy also prescribed that statues of the gods be cleansed with perfumed oils. In the Bible, Moses' 'holy anointing oil', which was to be kept strictly for religious purposes, was used to initiate Aaron and his sons into priesthood, a practice which continued from generation to generation. The Hebrews also used ointments in their temples and in coronation ceremonies, as recorded in the description of the anointing of David: 'Then Samuel took the horn of oil and anointed him in the midst of his brethren.'[3]

Consecrated perfume oils thus were an important element in initiation rituals or other emotionally charged events, because of their ability to inscribe on the memory a long-lasting impression, which could then be retrieved through association at a later date. Certain fragrances were also used in 'rites of passage' ceremonies to help dissolve conditioned psychological boundaries and open the psyche to transformation. A remnant of this tradition is still upheld in Britain today, the only nation in the world where the monarch is crowned with full Christian rites. Upon accession to the throne, the new king or queen is anointed with a 'coronation oil' at Westminster Abbey. This amber-coloured unguent consists of the essential oils of rose, orange blossom, jasmine and cinnamon, together with benzoin, musk, civet and ambergris in a sesame oil base. The recipe dates back to the seventeenth century – a vestige from the past when perfumes were themselves considered to be primarily sacred substances.

So the first perfumes, like incense, had a magico-religious significance and their employment and effects were predominantly of a therapeutic or psychological nature. Any object or person anointed with a consecrated oil was thereby sanctified and transformed. Perfume was not considered simply an adornment or luxury, but a vital necessity for everyday life, especially for the performance of sacred rituals. However, its other principal use in ancient civilizations, as confirmed by early texts and legends, was as a beauty aid or tool of seduction!

Religion, Sex and Perfume

> Poets quite rightly endow perfumes with the power
> to create a sweet intoxication in the soul.[4]

In India, the Hindu god Indra is always represented with his breast anointed with sandalwood oil, while the Hindu god of love, Kama, is shown with one of his five arrows tipped with jasmine. Divinity, sex and perfume were bound together in the oriental mind, since aromatics were recognized as contributing to the attainment of religious or sexual ecstasy. In Hindu and Buddhist Tantric practice, sex is seen as a means of spiritual realization and accomplishment through the dynamic exchange of male and female energy. In the Tantric 'Rite of the Five Essentials', jasmine oil is applied to the hands of the woman, patchouli to her neck and cheeks, amber to her breasts, spikenard to her hair, musk to the genital region, sandalwood to her thighs and saffron to her feet. Sandalwood oil is then applied to the man's forehead, neck, chest, navel, arms, thighs, genital region, hands and feet.

Likewise, in Chinese Taoist philosophy, sexuality is seen as a sacred art to be cultivated, since it represents the ultimate union of the primal cosmic forces, *yin* and *yang*. Many Indian, Chinese and Japanese practices, as well as certain pagan rites in the West (like that of the May pole), involve the worship of phallic statues or images of the female genitals as symbols of life and fertility. Such rituals sometimes involve offering or anointing the image with scented oil. The most famous sexual manual of all, the *Kama Sutra* or the *Kama Shastri*, 'The Scripture of Love', contains many references to aromatics. Here the sensual aspect of perfume is utilized in the art of love-making:

> ... the outer room, balmy with rich perfumes, should contain a bed, soft, agreeable to the sight, covered with a clean white cloth, low in the middle part, having garlands and bunches of flowers upon it, and a canopy over it, and two pillows, one at the top, another at the bottom. There should also be a sort of couch besides and at the head of this a sort of stool, on which should be placed the fragrant ointments for the night, as well as flowers ... and other fragrant substances.[5]

As in India and Egypt, the Greek mythologies attribute the origin and the use of perfumes to the Immortals. According to one legend, the human race derived its knowledge of them from the indiscretion of Aeone. Aeone was a nymph of Venus and Venus was the mistress of seduction, for which the use of perfumes was indispensable. Her temple altar was as sweetly scented as her body:

> She went away
> to Cyprus, and entered her fragrant
> temple at Paphos, where she had a precinct
> and a fragrant altar. After going inside

> she closed the bright doors, and the
> Graces gave her a bath, they oiled her
> with sacred olive oil, the kind that the
> gods always have on, that pleasant ambrosia
> that she was perfumed with.[6]

Divinity, sexuality and perfume are integrated in the image of the goddess Aphrodite hiding her nakedness behind a sprig of myrtle leaves. In Greek, the ancient word for myrtle is directly derived from the term 'perfume', so closely did they identify its fragrance with all that is beautiful and alluring. The fragrance of myrtle is still considered a potent aphrodisiac throughout Greece and the Middle East, where the freshly strewn leaves are used for scenting rooms. It is also used extensively as a bath preparation and in perfumery.

Likewise, in the Kore myth, it is while Persephone is picking spring flowers that she is abducted by Hades. Here, it is as if it was the heady scent of the flowers' fragrance which intoxicated her and transported her to another dimension – in this case the realm of the underworld. The Earth used 'a trick' of seduction, which she knew would be irresistible:

> Picking flowers,
> roses, and crocus
> and beautiful violets,
> in lush meadow,
> and iris, and hyacinth,
> narcissus even
> which Earth,
> as a trick,
> grew
> for this girl
> as a favour for
> Him Who Receives So Many.
> From its root
> it pushed up
> a hundred heads
> and a fragrance
> from its top
> making
> all the vast sky above
> smile...[7]

These flowers are all well-known aromatics: the fragrance of the crocus (saffron) was highly prized by the ancient Greeks, rose was considered to be an aphrodisiac, and iris and narcissus were thought to be narcotic.

Likewise, Homer records that when Circe set out to overcome Ulysses she employed powerful aromatic philtres and that Hera used perfumed oil to seduce Zeus in *The Iliad*.

Ancient Aphrodisiacs

But nowhere, perhaps, has the sensual lure of perfume been used to such effect as by Cleopatra. Queen Cleopatra was, like Venus herself, a mistress of seduction and well versed in the intoxicating effects of perfume. Even the sails of her barge, according to Shakespeare in *Anthony and Cleopatra*, were impregnated with a 'strange invisible perfume' which made the wind itself 'love sick'. During a banquet with Mark Anthony, Athenaeus records that the floors of the palace were strewn with rose petals to the depth of half a metre. Mark Antony could not resist such temptation – although the actual purpose of his encounter with the queen had initially been to question her about treachery to Rome!

Of course, the Romans were themselves no strangers to the power of perfume, renowned as they were for their hedonistic life-style. In the city of Rome particularly, the cult of perfumes was carried to extravagant extents, while in Capua a whole street was given over to perfumers.

According to Pliny, the Romans considered the use of perfumes one of the most honest pleasures of man, yet gradually scent also came to be associated with the orgiastic cults and lack of morality which were prevalent at the time. The philosophy of hedonism, which was established at the School of Cyrene by Aristippe (435–350 BC), a contemporary of Plato, further promoted the image of perfume as a self-indulgent, luxury item, an image which it has largely retained today.

A passion for powerful scents was also prevalent in the harems of old Constantinople. It is said of Mohammed that his sweat had the scent of roses, though he also singled out the aroma of musk as a favourite sexual stimulant. Perfumes of animal origin, such as musk or civet, naturally incite lust or 'impart energy to passion', since they are closely related to human physiological secretions. The strong Arab and

Turkish olfactory tradition is reflected in their love of heavy, musky, oriental perfumes, whose lingering scent still pervades their cities today. The Arabian fourteenth-century sexual treatise *The Perfumed Garden* of Shaykh Nefzawi gives a taste of the delight and power of perfume enjoyed by the Arabs, especially in relation to the way in which fragrance could be used for erotic purposes. In 'The Use of Perfumes in Coition: The History of Mocailama', it is said that:

> The use of perfumes, by man as well as by woman, excites to the act of copulation. The woman, inhaling the perfumes employed by the man, becomes intoxicated; and the use of scents has often proved a strong help to man, and assisted him in getting possession of a woman.[8]

The following advice on the art of seduction relates to the encounter between the prophetess Chedjâ el Temimia and Moicailama, an 'enemy of God' and one of the strongest competitors of Mohammed. Moicailama was successful in his overthrow of Chedjâ, who 'lost all presence of mind' under the influence of the aromas prepared for her ...

> Tomorrow morning erect outside the city a tent of coloured brocades, provided with silk furniture of all sorts. Fill the tent afterwards with a variety of different perfumes, amber, musk and all sorts of scents, as rose, orange flowers, jonquils, jessamine, hyacinth, carnation and other plants. This done, have then placed there several gold censers filled with green aloes, ambergris, *nedde* [this is a mixture of various perfumes, mainly benzoin and amber which are moulded into small cylinders and burnt upon coals] and so on. Then fix the hangings so that none of these perfumes can escape out of the tent. Then when you find the vapour strong enough to impregnate water, sit down on your throne, and send for the prophetess to come and see you in your tent, where she will be alone with you. When you are thus together there, and she inhales the perfumes, she will delight in the same, all her bones will be relaxed in a soft repose, and finally she will be swooning. When you see her thus far gone, ask her to grant you her favours; she will not hesitate to accord them.[9]

Among the Tunisian Bedouins, it is still customary for a newly wed couple to cover themselves with the pervasive scent of sarghuine before they first sleep together. Women from the Micronesian island of Nauru also perfume themselves copiously in preparation for a night of love.

They rub their bodies and hair with fragrant coconut oil and take steam baths using scented dakare bark. This rite is performed in secret.

Havelock Ellis also draws attention to the connection between sex and scent in Africa:

> When a woman of Swahili wishes to make herself desirable she anoints herself all over with fragrant ointments, sprinkles herself with rose water, puts perfume into her clothes, strews jasmine flowers on her body as well as binding them around her neck and waist.[10]

Similar practices are also common among South American natives. In the West, however, through its affinity with divinity and religion on the one hand and seduction and sex on the other, perfume came to be looked upon with an attitude of ambivalence that it still carries to a certain extent today. Is scent sacred or profane?

Scent: Sacred or Profane?

> It is difficult to guess which was the most potent source of the guilt that permeates modern Western mores, the Essenes in the desert of the Holy Land of the last century before Christ or the Puritans of modern and central Europe.[11]

Unlike the Orient, which has retained its original reverence and love of exotic perfumes, the West has at times outlawed the use of aromatics, due to their association with sexuality. This is due primarily to the influence of religious attitudes towards the body in the Western tradition. The ambiguity of the Christian view is evident from the earliest times, for although perfumes played an important part in Jewish religious life right up to the destruction of the Temple in AD 70, their secular use was initially associated with prostitution, sacred or otherwise. Jezebel's notoriety for using cosmetics – 'a painted Jezebel' – persists to this day as a symbol of vulgarity, while her familiarity with perfumes and aromatics associated her with pagan worship and the cult of Baal: 'What peace, so long as the whoredoms of thy mother Jezebel and her witchcrafts are so many?'[12]

It was Solomon who did most to put the use of perfumes on an acceptable basis. In the Old Testament, the 'Song of Songs' uses metaphors of the greatest sensuality and refinement to describe the act of love. Here, the body is revered and worshipped as a sacred temple and the pervasive scent of aromatics is referred to throughout to help bring to life the evocative sexual imagery:

> Your love is more delightful than wine;
> delicate is the fragrance of your perfume,
> your name is an oil poured out,
> and that is why the maidens love you …
> While the King rests in his own room
> my nard yields its perfume.
> My beloved is a sachet of myrrh
> Lying between my breasts.
> My Beloved is a cluster of henna flowers
> among the vines of Engedi.[13]

However, by the time the New Testament was written, the allure of perfume and the employment of scented unguents had come to be associated with depravity and indulgence. When Mary Magdalene anointed the feet of Jesus just before the Last Supper with a 'pound of ointment of spikenard very costly', Judas Iscariot asked, 'Why was not this ointment sold for three hundred pence and given to the poor?'[14] Christ legitimized Mary's action by giving it a sacred significance, yet the intimation remained that if a perfume was not intended specifically for religious use, it was, at best, superfluous. (Mary Magdalene became the patron saint of perfumers, based on her appreciation of the sweet smelling nard.)

Perfumes have been banned from use at various periods during history, yet such a step has never been maintained for long. In 1770 an Act was passed by the English Parliament that aimed at protecting those men who had been beguiled into matrimony by the use of scent or other types of 'witchcraft', by declaring such a marriage 'null and void'. The barbaric witch hunts and bleak Puritanism of Cromwell's reign did much to destroy the love of perfume and sensual pleasure altogether. But by the time of the Reformation, perfumes were back in full force. Charles II was especially fond of fragrance. Yet, even as recently as 1913, Dabney argued that:

> The use of perfumes from time immemorial has been a conscious or an unconscious attempt to stimulate lecherous thought, though in times of moral decay woman have, unfortunately, not been the only offenders.[15]

So, on the one hand, perfume is associated with spirituality, on the other with profanity. It is both the token of divinity and the tool of seduction. In the Christian depreciation of the body, perfume came to be seen as associated with temptation and sin. The instincts and their sensual demands were to be despised rather than heightened, for the sacred dimension within matter had been banished.

> Instinct guides the natural man in his physical world, but reason guides the civilized man in the social environment. Abandoning his animal existence, civilized man dulls the keenness of his sense of smell. However, by using his imagination he also expands it in a way not open to the savage.[16]

The degradation of the natural instincts was augmented by the seventeenth-century philosophy of Descartes, which defined man as a machine with reason at its helm. Yet to Rousseau, who held the senses in high esteem, odours not only influenced the purely physical drives, they also moved the imagination and stimulated aesthetic refinement:

> The sense of smell is the sense of imagination; giving a stronger tone to the nerves, it greatly disturbs the brain; which explains why it can arouse the amorous temperament momentarily, but eventually exhausts it.[17]

To the Greeks, too, aromatics were associated with all that was 'enthusiastic' and 'inspired' – the very word 'inspire' refers to the act of breathing in. There is a special relationship between scent and imagination not only because certain odours inspire passion and creativity, but because of the emotive imagery that perfumes can evoke. Ellis, in his classic work *Studies on the Psychology of Sex*, draws a sharp line between olfaction and the other senses:

> But smell with us has ceased to be a leading channel of intellectual curiosity. Personal odours do not, as vision does, give us information that is very largely intellectual; they make an appeal that is mainly of an intimate, emotional, imaginative character.[18]

Proust was inspired to write *A la Recherche du Temps Perdu* in response to the scent of madeleine biscuits reminiscent of his childhood. Goethe recounts how Schiller always kept a drawer full of rotten apples in his desk, because he found their scent inspirational. Both Zola, in *La Faute de l'Abbé Mouret*, and Baudelaire, in *Les Fleurs du Mal*, express delight in the rich imagery of odours, while the English poet Robert Herrick records the scent of his lovers with exquisite intensity. Indeed, fragrance is often used in love poetry because of its emotive quality. Of the five senses, smell is the most subtle, the most mysterious, being closest to the unconscious animal instincts and our ancestral nature.

In the West, as long as perfume is seen to elevate the spirit and cultivate refinement in the pursuit of beauty it is permissible. Thus, in the composition and use of modern perfumes, the age-old sexual message is overlaid with a restraint dictated by cultural conditioning, which leaves one wondering why anyone should wish to change their odour, 'to unconsciously reveal what they aim to hide'?[19]

Smell: The Secret Sense

The most mysterious, the most human thing, is smell.[20]

Without knowing it, people communicate sexual attraction to one another to a greater or lesser degree by scent. This has been recognized for thousands of years but it is only recently that the substances responsible have been given a name – 'pheromones', from the Greek for 'transfer' and 'excitement'. Of 200 separate compounds distinguishable in the normal body smells of men and women, androstenone, fatty acids, trimethylamine and isobutyraldehyde are the main human pheromones. Androstenone is the most important sexual messenger, with a scent similar to musk and sandalwood. It occurs naturally in sweat, tears, urine and hair (particularly genital hair), then travels by air to be picked up by the sensors in the nose. It is registered by that part of the brain concerned with smell, later to be finetuned by the rest of the intelligent cortex – yet a third of the population can't smell it!

In one study, carried out by Kirk-Smith and Booth[21] in a university dentist's waiting room, various chairs were sprayed with androstenone and then the choice of chairs used by patients was monitored by the receptionist. The results showed that whereas men tended to avoid or be oblivious to the odour, a significantly higher number of women chose scented chairs, even when the odorant concentration was applied at subliminal levels.

> A lot goes on under the surface. CAT scanning X-rays may show activity in the odour-related areas of the brain of a person who categorically denies perceiving a particular scent or flavour.[22]

According to Gary Schwartz of the University of Arizona, who has specifically studied the subliminal effects of scent, about 99 per cent of olfactory input is unconscious. Yet human beings are the most 'highly scented' of the apes, which suggests that they have a well developed scent communication system – whether they are aware of it or not. In the course of evolution, the human sense of smell has been downgraded in favour of the other senses, especially those of sight and hearing. In the West particularly, there has been a tremendous overloading on to the sense of sight – over 70 per cent of experience is processed visually. Why is this?

Freud believed that when humans began to walk on two legs, with 'nose raised from the ground', it brought about a change in the human experience of scent. He argued that a process of organic repression characterized the development of civilized man, which transformed the perceived quality of odours, including the smell of faeces, sweat and other sexual secretions, from pleasant to repulsive. What Freud failed to answer was why humans adopted the bipedal gait in the first place. In *The Scented Ape*, Michael Stoddard proposes that early man ceased to move about on four legs because exposure to sexual odours of other possible mates would be counter-productive to the preservation of the species:

> The adoption of a gregarious habit by man's ancestors probably during the Miocene epoch posed a threat to the pair bonds and that. . . there occurred some significant changes in the olfactory system which resulted in the odour clues associated with ovulation being rendered meaningless and even unpleasant.[23]

Stoddard argues that the maintenance of a stable pair bond was vital for the safety and well-being of their offspring, which require many years to reach maturity, and that slowly the sense of smell became less essential to survival. Seen in this context, the human adoption of the upright stance and changes in olfactory function was not so much a 'repression' as an 'evolved attribute of adaptive significance'. Nevertheless, a person's scent still plays an important role in human attraction or aversion. Women are especially sensitive to this, albeit often at an unconscious level. Each person has their own 'odourprint', as unique as a fingerprint. Among some north African tribes, a wife can instantly be divorced if she does not smell right!

In 1982, Preti, an organic chemist, and Cutler, a biologist, conducted a series of experiments to find out how humans responded to the smell of the opposite sex. In one test, a group of women who had irregular menstrual cycles was subjected three times a week to the underarm secretions of male donors, while another group was given a placebo. Within three-and-a-half months the first group had stabilized at an average cycle length of 28.3 days, while the second group averaged 41.2 days. Preti concluded that there must be something in the underarm region that affects the menstrual cycle, probably regulating hormones to ensure fertility, which seems to act like a primer pheromone.

> The latent possibilities of sexual allurement by olfaction which are inevitably embodied in the nervous structure we have inherited from our animal ancestors still remain ready to be called into play. They emerge prominently from time to time in exceptional and abnormal persons.[24]

This ability can be quite acute in some individuals, as Havelock Ellis suggests. Certainly, it has been noted that some types of neurotic conditions, such as schizophrenia, can often be accompanied by an acute hyper-sensitivity to smells – such individuals tend to be 'closer' to the unconscious than ordinary people. Additionally, the Native Americans, African tribesmen and Aborigine bushmen have retained a much higher olfactory ability than so-called 'civilized' peoples, who are more cut off from their instincts. Modern man has largely de-sensitized himself to the affects of odours, partly because they are seen as frivolous or of little consequence, but also because of the inherent underlying sexual connotation of certain fragrances.

Perfumes as Sexual Attractants

> Smells are forceful and erotic ... so they are looked on askance by our ethnic, which encourages restrained and rational behaviour.[25]

Nevertheless, the appeal of commercial perfumes still rests largely on the magnetic attraction that the wearer will supposedly have for members of the opposite sex. One perfume made by Jovan was actually called 'Andron', because it was said to have been made with minute quantities of andro-stenone and marketed as a sexual attractant. Humans have thus substituted their own alluring scent for the sexual odours of flowers and animals, such as those of the boar, musk deer, civet cat or beaver!

> The ingredients of perfumes may be summarized rather bluntly in the following manner: The top notes are made from the sexual secretion of flowers, produced to attract animals for the purposes of cross pollination and often formulated as mimics of the animals' own sex pheromones ... the middle notes are made from resinous materials which have odours not unlike those of sex steriods, while the base notes are mammalian sex attractants with distinctly urinous or faecal odour.[26]

Seen in this way, perfumes are little more then bottled sex pheromones! Although perfumes do perform a masking function, they also enhance and blend with the natural body odours. This accounts for why the same perfume can smell quite different, depending on who is wearing it.

While the top notes of a perfume create an initial impression, it is the base notes which contain the real message! Thus the purpose of using sex attractants in modern perfumes is to jog the ancient memory traces in the brain, and so in a 'sublime and vicarious manner'[27] reveal precisely what the 'artificial' fragrance helps to conceal. Yet such odours still have a strong and effective subliminal power despite the evolutionary suppression of the olfactory sense:

> The ambivalence of humankind towards the olfactory sense and odorous world results from this suppression – our memory traces, our olfactory vestiges are an Achilles' heel, a soft spot overlying a key to our deeper personalities which natural selection has inexplicably failed to patch ... our lack of mass odour culture is atavistic, reminding us of our evolutionary and biological relationships with our ancestors – creatures whose bones we can see in the museum cabinet but whose lives remain a mystery.[28]

Modern attitudes towards perfume and odour still largely remain ambivalent because they provide a subtle reminder of our common ancestral roots. However, in recent years, a general shift has been occurring in the sensory ratio towards the tactile and olfactory senses and the potential of scent is currently being re-evaluated. This seems to indicate an underlying reassessment of values and an attempt to reintegrate the 'feminine', 'earthy' or instinctual aspects of experience which have been repressed in the course of human evolution, especially in the West.[29]

There has also been a great deal of research carried out over the last few decades with regard to the effects of fragrance, as science comes to the realization that scent may indeed have a great deal to offer – and not just in the area of sex! The healing and regenerative powers of essential oils particularly are being reaffirmed, while the psychological effects of fragrance bring a 'message of hope' to all those suffering the stresses and strains of twentieth-century life.

> Floral earth, the sexual planet ... squeezed from the reproductive glands of plants and creatures, perfume, the smell of creation, a sign dramatically delivered to our senses of the Earth's regenerative powers – a message of hope and a message of pleasure...[30]

References

1. Agrippa, H. C., *La Philosophie Occulte*, 1531.
2. Shelmerdine, C. W., *The Perfume Industry of Mycenaean Pylos*, P. A. Forlag, 1985, p.57.
3. 1 Samuel 16: 13.
4. Cabanis, P. J. G., *Oeuvres Complètes*, Paris, 1956, p.228.
5. Cited in Tisserand, M., *Aromatherapy for Lovers*, Thorsons, 1993, p.31.
6. *The Homeric Hymns*, trans. Charles Boer.
7. Ibid.
8. Nefzawi, Shaykh, *The Perfumed Garden*, trans. Sir Richard Burton, Neville Spearman Ltd., 1963, p.79.
9. Ibid., p.83.
10. Cited in Carrington, H., *Perfumes: Their Sensual Lure and Charm*, Haldeman-Julius Publications, 1947, p.20.
11. Lake, M., *Scents and Sensuality*, Murray, 1989, Chapter 25.
12. 2 Kings 9: 22.
13. Song of Songs 1: 2–3 and 12–14.

14. John 12: 3–9.
15. Dabney, 1913, cited in Le Guèrer, A., *Scent: The Mysterious Power of Smell*, Chatto and Windus, 1993, p.169.
16. Ibid.
17. Cited ibid.
18. Stoddart, D. M., *The Scented Ape*, Cambridge University Press, 1990, p.128.
19. Lake, M., *Scents and Sensuality*, Murray, 1989, p.45.
20. Coco Chanel.
21. Kirk-Smith, Dr M., 'Human Olfactory Communication', Aroma '93 Conference at Sussex University.
22. Lake, op. cit., p.1.
23. Stoddart, op. cit, p.215.
24. Cited in Carrington, op. cit., p.21.
25. Howes, *Vegetarian Times*, October 1992, p.97.
26. Stoddart, op. cit., p.13.
27. Ibid.
28. Dodd, G. H. and Van Toller, S., *Perfumery: The Psychology and Biology of Fragrance I*, Chapman and Hall, 1990, p.17.
29. See Steele, J., 'The Fragrance of the Goddess' in *Aromatherapy Quarterly*, Summer 1990, p.10.
30. Robbins, Tom, 'Jitterbug Perfume', cited in Lake, M., op. cit., p.32.

five 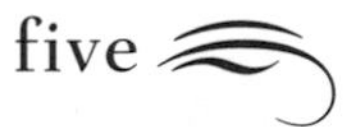

Psycho-Aromatherapy

Hence do I likewise minister perfume
Unto the neighbour brain, perfume of force,
To cleanse your head, and make your fancy bright,
To refine wit and sharp invention
And strengthen memory: from whence it came
That old devotion, incense did ordain
To make man's spirit more apt for things divine ...

A. Brewer, *Lingua or The Combat of the Tongue and the Five Senses*, Act IV, Scene 5, c.1600.

The psychological benefits of fragrance have been recognized for hundreds of years in the West, while herbs have been used for their specific effects by so-called 'primitive' peoples since the dawn of civilization. There is no doubt that in the past natural aromatic substances have been employed successfully for their sedative, stimulating, hallucinogenic, sexually arousing or anaesthetising effects, yet as Michael Stoddard points out in *The Scented Ape*:

> A thorough and exhaustive investigation of the psychotropic action of essential oils is long overdue and is needed to convince sceptics of the benefits of aromatherapy and to provide a clear explanation for the psychosomatic foundations for aromatherapy.[1]

Essential oils, which constitute the odiferous part of a plant, are the tools of the modern practice known as 'aromatherapy', which, by means of massage, baths, vaporization, etc., utilizes their vital healing properties. Aromatherapy is a holistic type of treatment based on psychosomatic principles because it takes the physical, emotional and mental needs of the individual into consideration.

Psycho-aromatherapy, which focuses on the psychological potential of essential oils, concerns itself primarily with the effects of fragrance, since it has been found that psychotherapeutic results can be obtained more easily and quickly through smell than through any other method. However, massage can also be very beneficial, especially for emotional problems and stress related conditions, because it combines inhalation with the healing effects of touch. Aromatic bathing is also valuable in this context, because it combines scent with relaxation, as well as promoting absorption of the essential oils through the skin. In psycho-aromatherapy, the physiological effects of essential oils on the nervous system are combined with the individual's emotional or psychological reaction to their aroma, both aspects working together in psychosomatic unity. Thus the practice of pyscho-aromatherapy, while concentrating on the benefits of fragrance, actually embraces a wide variety of different methods and techniques which can be employed at home as well as in a professional context.

But how exactly does the olfactory system operate, and what other processes are involved in the way aromatics affect the physiological and psychological state of an individual? In understanding such questions, it is valuable to juxtapose past evidence with modern research, so as to build up a comprehensive picture of the therapeutic potential of natural aromatics.

The Olfactory Process

When we smell a rose, its sweet fragrance enters into our nose with our breath. Its scent is made up of minute aromatic molecules or 'energy particles', each of which has a specific shape. Located at the top and on both sides of the upper nasal cavity is the *olfactory epithelium*, which is covered with a thin layer of mucus. Once in the nose, the aromatic molecules migrate through the mucus to the underlying tissue of about 10 million olfactory nerve cells. Each nerve cell carries a bundle of tiny hairs or *cilia* equipped with different receptor cells to fit each aromatic molecule shape, like a key in a lock. These receptors are extremely sensitive and capable of carrying a vast amount of information. The human nose can detect up to 10,000 different odours at minute concentrations – vanilla, for example, can be detected at concentration levels of .00000000762 grains per cubic inch.

The receptors then transmit the odour along the nerve fibres, in the form of electrical impulses, to the *olfactory bulb*, which in turn passes the stimulus to other relevant parts of the brain. This chemo-sensory information is then translated into physiological and behavioural effects, and finally, by comparison with memory contents, into a conscious olfactory experience. The scent of a rose, for example, passes directly to the *limbic system* or the pre-frontal part of the brain, where past memories associated with the fragrance are evoked immediately. The limbic system, where feelings and instincts are recorded, was already well developed in our ancestors, since in earlier times humans depended on their sense of smell for survival. It was only later that 'civilized' man came to depend on the more recently evolved *cerebral cortex,* which filters incoming information as well as governing speech and intellectual knowledge.

It is only within the last 20 years that scientists have begun to understand how our sense of smell works – although there is still much to be explained. In the early 1980s a biologist named Pasquale Graziadei observed that the olfactory cells 'were undergoing a phenomenal regeneration', and that only mature cells were actually responding to specific odours and sending meaningful messages to the brain. According to Graziadei, 'each odor seems to stimulate the nerve cells in a unique pattern within the nose' and these patterns have had a pivotal role in the evolution of man:

> It looks like the forebrain literally develops under the influence of the nose ... For instance, human babies born with anencephaly – a disorder in which the brain is missing – also lack a nose. Without the nose, the brain might suffer severely in its development.[2]

In animals, smell provides the primary motivation for the basic behaviour of approach and avoidance, and the suggestion is that olfaction may still be the foundation of emotional response in the human realm. Unlike visual or oral stimuli, which are processed by the cerebral cortex, odours pass straight to the olfactory bulb where they are given an immediate 'feeling' value. This also accounts for why we can be affected by odours without even being conscious of the fact – the information has bypassed the cerebral cortex and entered directly into the innermost 'control centres' of the limbic system.

> Odor stimuli in the limbic system or olfactory brain release neurotransmitters – among them encephaline, endorphins, serotonin, and noradrenaline. Encephaline reduces pain, produces pleasant euphoric sensations, and creates a feeling of well-being. Endorphins also reduce pain, stimulate sexual feelings, and produce a sense of well-being. Serotonin helps relax and calm, and noradrenaline acts as a stimulant that helps keep you awake. Within the limbic system resides the regulatory mechanism of our highly explosive inner life, the secret core of our being. Here is the seat of our sexuality, the impulses of attraction and aversion, our motivation and our moods, our memory and creativity, as well as our autonomic nervous system.[3]

These complex nervous and hormonal activities are orchestrated by the limbic system via the hypothalamus. Thus emotional or instinctual reactions registered by the limbic system are translated into physical responses, such as the 'fight or flight' mechanism, sexual impulses or the expression of pleasure. Certain scents can even affect the regulation of the autonomic nervous system, which is not usually subject to conscious influence, by bringing about changes in the functioning of the heartbeat, the depth of breathing or the digestive processes. And since odours touch the subconscious level, which is a limitless resource of creative impulses, this also helps to explain why certain scents can stimulate the imagination and evoke inspiration.

Having been picked up by the limbic system, the aromatic molecules continue their journey towards the lungs, where they eventually pass through the delicate moist walls of the alveoli and into the blood capillaries. From the capillaries, the tiny molecules are conveyed to the heart and the circulatory system, which means they have access to all the organs and systems of the body. The psychological effect of the scent on the mind and emotions is thus combined with a physiological action on the body. Thus in odour perception, it could be said that there are two distinct dimensions involved – the physio-chemical/physiological dimension and the psycho-logical/emotional dimension:

> Characteristically, odour and fragrance are perceived as having two main types of reaction, namely, physiological and psychological. The former acts directly on the body, while the latter affects the mind through the brain.[4]

The Physiological Effect of Fragrance on the Nervous System, especially in Relation to Depression and Anxiety

> How reviving and pleasing some scents of flowers are is obvious to all; and what great virtues they may have in diseases, especially of the head, may easily be conjectured by any thinking man … I remember that, when walking in a long gallery of the Indian House in Amsterdam, where vast quantities of mace, cloves and nutmegs were kept in great open chests, I found something so reviving in the perfumed air that I took notice of it to the company with me, which was a great deal, and they were all sensible of the same effect … the use of scents is not practised in modern physic but might be carried out with advantage, seeing that some smells are so depressing and others so reviving and inspiring.[5]

So wrote Sir William Temple in 1690 in his *Essay on Health and Long Life*. Dr W. S. Watson had also noted the exhilarating effect of odours, especially on the mentally ill, which he reported in the *Medical Press and Circular* of Great Britain, 1875. Almost 100 years later, in his book *In Search of Perfumes Lost*, Prof. Rovesti drew attention once more to the potential of fragrance in the treatment of psychological disorders, especially depression and anxiety:

> The possibility of contributing new therapeutic solutions to these two now very common psychoneuroses is therefore of notable interest, especially in view of the fact that the essential oils used in aromatherapy, if in appropriate doses and application, are harmless to the organism and do not give rise to any of the disturbances caused by chemical drugs. It must be said that ever since the remotest times the fumigations of certain aromatic plants have been employed as tranquillizers and antispasmodics in cases of erethism [irritability] and of high nervous tension and conversely as excitants against fainting fits and depressive states.[6]

Indeed, the therapeutic potential of scent has been recognized for thousands of years in the West without being fully utilized. It is only this century that systematic research has been carried out in this area, with very promising results.

In the early 1920s, two Italian doctors, Giovanni Gatti and Renato Cayola, published a report, *The Action of Essences on the Nervous System*, in which they explored the effects of various essential oils on the two opposing states of anxiety and depression. The experiments were conducted using either a cotton-wool pad impregnated with an essential oil and applied to the face with a mask or an aromatic solution which was sprayed into the surrounding air and then inhaled. The doctors then measured changes in the pulse rate, blood circulation and depth of breathing.

Their results demonstrated that scents can exert an influence on the brain very quickly, since the inhalation method brought about an almost immediate effect, in contrast to the oral administration, where the essential oils were absorbed slowly via the digestive system. The essential oils which they identified as sedatives – and therefore of use in anxiety states – included chamomile, melissa, neroli, petitgrain, opoponax, asafoetida and valerian. Stimulating essences, on the other hand, useful in the treatment of depression, included angelica, cardamom, lemon, fennel, cinnamon, clove and ylang ylang (an aphrodisiac). The researchers also noted that some essences were stimulating in small doses, but sedative in larger amounts (much like wine!) They concluded that:

> The sense of smell has, by reflex action, an enormous influence on the function of the central nervous system.[7]

Then in 1937 Gattefossé published his *Aromathérapie*, the book which gave the modern practice of aromatherapy its name and which in many ways initiated the revival of using essential oils for healing purposes. In the section 'Action of Essences on the Nervous System', Gattefossé mentions the following oils as having a significant effect on the nervous functions: hawthorn, heliotrope, vanilla, cajuput, bay laurel, neroli, melissa and valerian have a tranquillizing effect, of value in hysterical and hypertensive conditions; borneol, angelica (at low doses) and savory (at low doses) are stimulating; clove, sage, myrtle and rose activate the sexual centres, while camphor, calamus and asafoetida have the opposite effect.

Dr Jean Valnet enhanced the medical status of essential oils through his work as a doctor during the Second World War and by his successful application of aromatics in the treatment of psychiatric patients between the 1950s and 1970s, the results of which he published in

The Practice of Aromatherapy (1980). He suggests that most essences are stimulants, including pine, borneol, geranium, basil, sage, savory, rosemary and lemon. On the other hand, lavender, lemongrass, marjoram, cypress and anise have anti-spasmodic properties. Onion, cinnamon, borneol, savory and ylang ylang stimulate the sexual faculties, whereas camphor has anaphrodisiac qualities.

Research in this field was then taken up by Prof. Paolo Rovesti of Milan University in the 1970s. He measured the restorative effect of pure essential oils on patients suffering from hysteria or nervous depression, using either oral administration or inhalation. Among the anxiety relieving essences which he found to be effective were bergamot, lime, neroli, petitgrain, lavender, marjoram, violet leaf, rose, cypress and opoponax. Against depressive states he utilized lemon, orange, verbena, jasmine, ylang ylang and sandalwood.

According to Rovesti, a blend of different oils is even more likely to have a positive therapeutic effect than individual essences because aromatic mixtures are generally perceived as being more pleasant. Since the brain tends to reject unpleasant odours,[8] they do not gain the same type of access to the central nervous system as those which are aesthetically pleasing. Therefore, for example, even if an oil has been found to have a definite sedative effect, it may not be therapeutically useful because of its unpleasant smell. Rovesti concluded that aesthetic considerations were thus very important in choosing the correct fragrance for therapeutic use.

Several trials have also been carried out regarding the sedative effect of essential oils on animals. Based on the results of these tests, all the following oils were found to result in a general depressional reduction in spontaneous movement: asafoetida, calamus, carrot seed, chamomile, clary sage, geranium, lavender, marjoram, melissa, rose, taget, valerian and yarrow. Several incense materials were also subjected to testing and here it was found that small amounts were distinctly stimulating while large amounts were often sedative. A further clinical study into the psychological effects of chamomile oil was also carried out recently at Cambridge University and the University of North Wales. This confirmed the oil's soothing effect on the nervous system of humans.

The Brain's Response to Fragrance

The first systematic study into the effect of fragrance on the brain was carried out by Moncrieff in 1962 using an EEG machine (an electroencephalogram). An EEG machine monitors brainwave patterns: an increase in alpha activity indicates relaxation, while an increase in beta activity shows stimulation. Moncrieff carried out two studies in which he recorded the brain's response to 17 different natural odours. He found that odours were indeed able to significantly influence the EEG levels. This discovery set the tone for later developments.

In 1979, John Steele carried out some preliminary experiments using the 'mind-mirror', a portable multi-channel EEG to evaluate the effects of various essential oils on the brain's rhythm patterns. The 'mind-mirror' is especially useful in researching altered states of consciousness. This led to further studies:

> As predicted, the cephalic oils (which stimulate mental clarity and memory) such as basil, rosemary, black pepper and cardamom, induced beta predominant patterns. Beta brain rhythms (38–13 Hertz) are correlated with aroused attention and alertness. At the other end of the spectrum, the floral antidepressant euphorics such as orange flower (neroli), jasmine and rose induced an unusual amount of delta rhythms (4–.75 Hertz) with some alpha (12–8 Hertz) and theta (7–5 Hertz) present. These slower frequencies indicate a quieting of mental chatter (alpha), with the mind going into reverie and intuitive flashes (theta and delta).[9]

Orange flower was especially relaxing. Other oils tested were lavender, geranium, cedarwood and lemongrass.

Then in the 1970s, Prof. Torii of Toho University, Japan, initiated a research programme aimed at specifically distinguishing between those oils which have a sedative effect on the nervous system and those which have a stimulating effect. During each experiment, the subject had electrodes attached to their scalp which showed their 'normal' EEG trace. The measuring device used was the CNV (contingent negative variation) curve, an electrical brainwave pattern created by anticipation.

True to expectation, initial studies showed that lavender suppressed the EEG trace, while jasmine increased it – in other words, lavender had a sedative effect and jasmine a stimulating one. A further 17 oils

The Effects of Essential Oils on the Nervous System

Sedative (anxiety)	*Stimulating (depression)*	*Aphrodisiac*
anise	angelica	borneol
bay	basil	cinnamon
bergamot	borneol	clove
cajeput	cardamom	myrtle
calamus	cinnamon	onion
carrot seed	clove	rose
chamomile	fennel	sage
clary sage	geranium	savory
cypress	jasmine	ylang ylang
geranium	lemon	
hawthorn	orange	***Anaphrodisiac***
heliotrope	pine	asafoetida
lavender	rosemary	calamus
lemongrass	sandalwood	camphor
lime	sage	
marjoram	savory	
melissa	verbena	
neroli	ylang ylang	
opopanax		
petitgrain		
rose		
taget		
vanilla		
violet leaf		
valerian		
yarrow		

Comprehensive Table of Stimulating and Sedative Essences (based on EEG material)

Sedative	*Stimulant*
bergamot	basil
bois de rose	bois de rose
chamomile	clove
geranium	geranium
lavender	jasmine
lemon	lemongrass
marjoram	neroli
sandalwood	patchouli
valerian	peppermint
	rose
	sage
	valerian
	ylang ylang

were tested by Torii altogether using CNV and of these, geranium and rosewood were shown to be either stimulating or sedative, as was valerian to a lesser extent! Such oils were capable of producing either one response or the other depending on the state of the individual. In aromatherapy these oils are known as 'adaptogens' and are said to be 'balancing' in effect, that is, they can have a restorative effect on listless or depressed patients as well as on those prone to hyperactivity or agitation.

It is clear from the results that some of the CNV traces on individual oils were contrary to expectation. Neroli and rose, for example, which are usually considered to be sedative oils, were shown to have a stimulating effect on brainwave activity. Lemon and sandalwood, on the other hand, which are often thought to be stimulating oils, both showed a marked sedative effect. Sage, surprisingly, made very little impact on the CNV trace at all, but was slightly stimulating. Similar results were also obtained by Sugano in his work using EEG, CNV and microvibration (MV) – a mechanism which measures muscle tension. He found that lavender and orange decreased muscle tension, while jasmine increased it. His EEG readings indicated that lavender, sandalwood, musk, eucalyptus and terpene compounds (forest smells) all increased alpha activity – in other words they all encouraged a relaxed state of mind, as in meditation. On the other hand, he found that eucalyptus depressed the CNV reading, while lavender, sandalwood and musk increased it. He concludes by recommending lavender or rose for release from stress, and jasmine and camphor for depression.

The divergence of opinion on whether oils such as rose or neroli are stimulating or sedative in effect may be due to a variety of factors. Gattefossé and Sugano both noted that results can vary or change according to concentration levels: 'Angelica essence at low doses stimulates the brain, but at high doses it becomes a narcotic.'[10]

In addition, it is quite feasible to assume that some oils may simultaneously stimulate brain activity whilst sedating other parts of the nervous system – or vice versa. With regard to rose oil, for example, Gattefossé mentions that according to Dr Marceval, rose essence stimulates the sexual centres and acts as an aphrodisiac (especially rose maroc), but he also cites F. Grégoire's work on frog hearts, in which he demonstrates that rose, like 'neroli essence and orangeflower water are tranquillisers which slow the heartbeat substantially'.[11] This tends to suggest that while neroli and rose essence do indeed stimulate the brain and uplift the spirits, at the same time they reduce the heartbeat and the blood pressure and soothe the nerves.

Research into the effect of different odours on mood has also shown that stimulation and relaxation are not mutually exclusive states. In this context, neroli and rose could be said to be essential oils which, like lemon and sandalwood, increase both stimulation and relaxation levels.

The actual interpretation of EEG studies is also made more complicated by the relative contribution of direct and indirect odour effects on a subject's behaviour and neurophysiology:

> Direct effects are non-cognitive in nature and are due to direct stimulation of the olfactory tract and other related brain structures ... indirect odour effects refer to those central nervous system changes resulting from cognitive activity related to the information conveyed by the odour.[12]

In a recent experiment[13] carried out by the International Flavors & Fragrance Inc., a commercial body who became interested in aromatherapy in the early 1980s, subjects were connected to a EEG machine which registered the brain's response to the scents of jasmine or lavender with a predictable result – the former showing a stimulating effect and the latter a sedative one. Later on, however, the subjects were again subjected to a combination of these two scents, but were purposely given contradictory information about what they were smelling. Here it was found that the subjects' CNV traces were affected by their beliefs and thoughts about the stimulus – which contradicted the earlier result. The recent work of Knasko (1990) has also demonstrated that even feigned environmental odours can alter mood and levels of stimulation – in other words, a mental idea can override a physical phenomenon. Such results indicate that in assessing the effects of a fragrance there are many other factors to be taken into consideration – especially when they are 'tainted' by indirect or cognitive information.

Van Toller and Kobal[14] also embarked on a study of brain function during olfactory stimulation and the effects of fragrance on the two sides of the brain: the right-hand side which deals with imagination, emotion and aesthetic awareness, and the left-hand side which is more concerned with reasoning, words and logic. Under normal conditions, both sides work harmoniously to integrate all incoming data, yet the researchers observed that when a perfume described as 'pleasant' was inhaled, a wave of electrical activity was initiated in the right hemisphere and then spread to parts of the left, presumably when the stimulus was integrated.

They also found that during the perception of an odour, the left-hand side of the brain could obscure what was happening on the right if thought processes – such as trying to name the scent or qualify it in some way – overrode the aesthetic or emotional reaction. The cognitive part of the brain was also found to intercede in an emotional response, if it deemed it inappropriate, and could even cancel out the hedonistic experience entirely.

These results confirm that brainwave activity is far more complex than was initially thought and the effect of an odour is ultimately dependent on what is going on within the mind of the subject. Although it is true to say that certain scents do tend to produce specific physical effects which are common to all people – stimulating or relaxing, pleasant or unpleasant – subjective psychological factors can override the more objective physiological response or at least colour the individual's reaction. Thus, even using sophisticated equipment, it is still difficult to qualify accurately the properties of a given odour or predict an individual's response to it, because of the psychological factors involved.

In agreement with the results of these reports, at the Psychology of Perfumery Conference 1991, it was generally accepted that 'while pharmacological effects may be very similar from one person to another, psychological effects are bound to be different'.[15] In other words, although the physiological and physio-chemical response may be predicted, the emotional or psychological reaction cannot. In the final analysis, the effect of an odour on an individual is therefore dependent on a number of individual factors, including:

1) how the odour was applied
2) how much was applied (concentration levels)
3) the circumstances in which it was applied
4) the person to whom it was applied (age, sex, personality type)
5) what mood they were in to start with
6) what previous associations they may have with the odour
7) anosmia or inability to smell (certain scents)
8) expectations or thoughts about the odour

The Psychological Dimension: Emotion and the Sense of Smell

> Perhaps no topic in the psychology of olfaction is of greater interest to both the general public and aroma researchers than the relationship between smell and emotion.[16]

Many illnesses could be said to be rooted in the mind, in a person's negative outlook or underlying fears. Mental states such as anxiety,

The Mind/Body Interaction

Mind/Psyche	***Smell***	***Body***
Anxiety/Confidence	<<<<<<<<>>>>>>>>>	Heart Rate
Stress/Relaxation		Breathing Rate
Irritation/Equilibrium		Muscle Tone

irritation or anger cause physical changes in the body, including an increase in heart rate, breathing and muscle tone. Complaints such as diarrhoea, asthma and hypertension are often directly related to mental disturbances. Stress and mental unrest, which are at the root of so much of our twentieth-century disease, eventually have a degenerative effect on the entire organism. The role of emotion has tended to be downplayed in our society, but this is beginning to change – the psychosomatic foundations of disease are being increasingly accepted in contemporary medical practice. The influence of emotion and mood is significant because 'how you feel can determine what you think, perceive, remember, and ultimately how you behave'.[17]

Since the body and mind are intrinsically related, a change in the emotional or psychological disposition of an individual can have dramatic results on their health as a whole. And since the limbic system, the emotional 'control centre' of the brain, is especially susceptible to the effects of fragrance, it is possible to heighten or influence the underlying disposition or attitude of a person by subjecting them to certain scents. Odours which carry a positive association, for example, can help to bring about a change of attitude by allowing the individual to re-experience pleasure or joy. This is one of the basic premises underlying the use of incense in ritual and religious practice, where the familiar scent of the incense helps to bring about, through repetition, a receptive and uplifted state of mind. Odours are especially potent in their influence when they are used for such purposes, because they largely operate on a subconscious or subliminal level, and have direct access to the emotional centres of the brain without experiencing the interference of thought processes:

> Using perfumes as fumigations in ritual therefore provides us with direct access to pre-programmed emotional states.[18]

In a recent experiment,[19] it was shown conclusively that an odour can be paired with a specific emotional response and that the emotional state can be re-evoked when the odour is reintroduced at a later date. The experiment involved a negative emotional response to an odour, but a positive association would operate in the same manner – perhaps to an even greater extent.

J. R. King has also found that some fragrances can be very effective in promoting relaxation, not only because of their sedative properties or pleasant associations, but also because they by-pass the critical faculties of the mind that can actually interfere with the success of this type of work. He has utilized a seaside fragrance in his relaxation studies, because of its widespread positive associations, although he points out that if it is then used to counteract negative moods in stressful situations, 'such a fragrance would be best used sparingly and for brief periods, to preserve its value as a conditioned stimulus'.[20]

To test the hypothesis that emotions and smell are fundamentally related Howard Ehrlichman of the City University of New York isolated subjects in a bare darkish room and then wafted pleasant and unpleasant odours into the air. In preliminary tests he found that the scent of almond stimulated pleasant memories in his subjects, while the odour of pyridine (like urine) provoked unhappy memories. Ehrlichman concluded:

> ... the experience of odor and the experience of emotion are in some basic, physiological way the same. Molecules of odor seem to be stimulating the same brain centres that signal the drives towards or away, which underlie almost all human emotion.[21]

There is also a reciprocal relationship between stress and scent, that is, certain smells, especially those with pheromonal potential, can cause a stress reaction and vice versa. Animals are particularly sensitive to this phenomenon and the smell of fear or disease can sometimes be picked up by humans with a trained nose. Happiness and good health also have their characteristic smell! At Yale University, the psychobiologist

Gary Schwartz began to research the effects of fragrance on stress using a combination of methods, including bio-feedback. He wired his subjects for measurements of blood pressure, muscle tension and skin temperature, then, after asking them a series of stressful questions, he exposed them to the scent of 1) an apple; 2) a spice; 3) a spicy apple. Although all three fragrances relaxed the subjects, the spiced apple fragrance was the most effective at reducing blood pressure and general stress levels. Subsequent research has shown that food smells are especially effective at inducing a feeling of well-being and relaxation, which may help to account for the success of the spicy apple fragrance. As Schwartz himself points out:

> Scents entering the nose might be absorbed by the bloodstream, exerting a chemical effect. At a more psycho-biological level, when we savor a pleasant fragrance, we take deeper and slower breaths, relaxing our respiratory pattern much as we do in meditation. The olfactory input might also serve as a distracter, focusing our attention on the scent or inducing positive memories and emotions.[22]

Mind, Mood and Memory

> Ah, these jasmines, these white jasmines!
> I seem to remember the first day when I
> filled my hands with these jasmines, these
> white jasmines.
> I have loved the sunlight, the sky and the
> green earth;
> I have heard the liquid murmur of the
> river through the darkness of midnight …
> Yet my heart is sweet with the memory
> of the first fresh jasmines that filled my hands
> when I was a child.[23]

There is no doubt that certain scents can evoke powerful personal memories and that they often tend to take on an individual significance connected with a particular childhood experience. The French psychoanalyst André Virel used odours to help bring forth forgotten or hidden memories in his clients. Odours can also be associated with specific feelings about a given person or place – the word 'atmosphere' is even derived from the Greek *atmos,* meaning 'vapour', showing the link between odour and mood. In a universal phenomenon called 'olfactory-evoked recall', a certain smell brings back a memory from the past, often together with a vivid visual image and a positive mood state. As in the poem 'The First Jasmines', a feeling of nostalgia can be induced with the greatest of ease through a remembered smell, perhaps more so than through the other senses, as Rudyard Kipling noted: 'Smells are surer than sights or sounds to make your heartstrings crack.'[24]

In 1985, the International Flavors & Fragrances Inc. instituted an 'Aroma Science' programme whose aim was to assess the effects of aromatics on subjective mood states using both physiological and psychological means. Physiological reactions were measured using galvanic skin response, skin temperature, muscle tension, heart rate, respiration and, especially, blood pressure. Psychological responses to specific odours were recorded by subjective self-reports.

Eight mood categories were used in a series of experiments in which various 'living flower' fragrances were given a 'mood profile' by a panel of 35–50 women. The eight mood categories were those usually employed in mood research studies carried out throughout the world, i.e. stimulation, sensuality, happiness, relaxation, apathy, depression, irritation and stress. During the test, muguet, osmanthus, Douglas fir and hyacinth were each judged according to their ability both to increase feelings of well-being and to decrease negative moods. Muguet was found to increase happiness, relaxation and stimulation while reducing irritation, depression and apathy; osmanthus increased happiness and stimulation while reducing all four negative mood categories; Douglas fir increased happiness and relaxation while reducing all four negative mood categories; and hyacinth increased all four positive mood categories while at the same time reducing all four negative ones.

The results demonstrate that fragrances can indeed have a significant effect on mood and that different scents tend to induce specific reactions – subject to individual experience. It is also apparent from the reports that relaxation and stimulation are not mutually exclusive mood states – a fact that researchers have been aware of for years. A fragrance which increases both stimulation and relaxation could be said to bring about a heightened sense of calm together with an increase in awareness and energy, in other words, a state of 'calm vitality'. Many essential oils could be said to have this property.

Having spent many years researching the effects of fragrance on mood, the IFF were led to the following observations:

1) That fragrance-evoked mood changes are small, but beneficial to our well-being.

2) That fragrance can be used to reduce the stress response in humans, but its physiological effects on a non-stressed subject are minimal and difficult to measure. Nutmeg, for example, was found to induce a marked reduction in the blood pressure of subjects under stress, yet exhibited no stress-reducing or relaxing effects when the subject was already at ease.

3) Pleasant odours were found particularly to enhance creative performance, help induce a positive evaluation of people or situations and elicit happy memories. By contrast, unpleasant odours tended to stimulate unpleasant thoughts and mood states.[25]

Subsequent research into the effects of odour on mood by Ehrlichman and Bastone (see 'The Use of Odour in the Study of Emotion') has enlarged upon the above results. In one study, which again included muguet, the mood scales sleepy/alert, annoyed/pleased, depressed/excited, tense/relaxed and disgusted/delighted were used. The results of these tests indicate that:

> The most consistent effects seem to be on general scales such as pleasant–unpleasant, annoyed–pleased or good–bad mood, whereas results for the mood adjective list (MACL), which assesses specific mood states (such as sadness, fear and anger), have been less supportive.[26]

The Persuasive Power of Fragrance

> Odours have a power of persuasion stronger than that of words, appearances, emotions or will. The persuasive power of an odour cannot be fended off, it enters into us like breath into our lungs, it fills us up, imbues us totally. There is no remedy for it.[27]

The power of fragrance is given great credence in the imaginative modern novel already mentioned – *Perfume: The Story of a Murderer* by

Patrick Süskind. In this book the central character Grenouille uses his remarkable olfactory talent as a means of controlling people, of duping them and exploiting them: to him it becomes a tool of power. The greatest secret is that the people do not even know that they are being tricked, because each perfume Grenouille concocts acts upon them in an unconscious manner, exuding a subtle 'hidden' magic.

> Under the sway of the odour, but without their being aware of it, people's facial expressions, their airs, their emotions were altered.[28]

This is the power of perfume: we are all influenced by odours in our daily lives, in our relationships, our moods, our preferences, our fantasies and our feelings, yet we are often unaware of it! This is because our sense of smell operates largely on an unconscious level, conditioning our behaviour unknowingly. Even when their concentration level is so weak that they are below the threshold of consciousness, odours still affect our moods subconsciously. This suggests that they have more influence over our decisions and judgements than we may like to imagine.

> So subtle is it, indeed, that I am persuaded its stimuli may, on occasion, not emerge into consciousness at all. They remain below the threshold. So that although subjected to their influence, we may remain ignorant of the cause of that influence. For smell often operates powerfully, not only surreptitiously enriching and invigorating the mental impression of an event, but also in directing at times the flow of ideas into some particular channel independent of the will.[29]

Indeed, one of the main difficulties in assessing the psychological effects of fragrance is the very fact that odour perception often remains at a subconscious level, as Maurice Thiboud points out:

> The great majority of psychological studies on odour response deal with the conscious processing of olfactory information, despite the fact that an argument can be made for odour perception being a phenomena largely at the periphery of conscious thought, only marginally accessible to self awareness.[30]

Future olfactory studies may indeed be more successful and conclusive if they are carried out without the subjects knowing what is going on!

But to what extent is it actually possible to control or condition another person's response to a particular aroma? Zoologist Michael Stoddard asserts that although there is no odour capable of inducing a systematic behaviour in man, it is nevertheless possible that we are still subconsciously manipulated by odours. Since the sexual and social instincts of humans are no longer governed by scent signals, as they are in other mammals, odours do not cause overt changes in human sexual or emotional behaviour; rather, they create changes in mood or feeling states, often at a subliminal level:

> ... in contrast to strong emotions, these feeling [mood] states do not interrupt our thoughts, but subtly colour and redirect them often without our notice.[31]

Yet it is because scents influence us largely unwittingly that they have such great psychological potential, for better or for worse ... Indeed, one reason for the Puritans' suspicion and rejection of perfumes was that in them they sensed a form of deception. There is more than a grain of truth in this, for scents certainly do have this potential. Seen in this context, it is clear that there is a need to distinguish between the beneficial and the insidious use of scent. This depends entirely on the motivation or purpose for its use.

At present there is a great deal of medical interest in the potential use of aromas for their psychological effects, and on this basis, Dodd and Van Toller have proposed the word 'osmotherapy' specifically to describe the utilization of scents, both natural and artificial, for therapeutic purposes.[32] Fragrance, for example, has been found to be an ideal candidate for use in relaxation work, not least because it directly targets the 'inner' mind and by-passes any critical interference by the verbal, conscious mind. The scientific establishment has also shown an increased interest in the role of scent, and the Fragrance Research Foundation in New York have in recent years coined the term 'aromachology' to describe the study and use of natural or synthetic odours in this field. However, both 'osmotherapy' and 'aromachology' are quite distinct from psycho-aromatherapy, in that the latter employs only natural fragrances derived from pure botanical sources within a 'holistic' therapeutic framework and also uses other methods of treatment apart from inhalation.

The current commercial trend is also moving towards a rapid increase in the utilization of fragrance as a marketing tool. In a trial test using fragranced shoes,[33] it was shown that customers were attracted to the scented items in preference to non-scented items – even if they did not know why. This is a matter of some concern, especially if the odour is released at subliminal levels beneath the conscious threshold, since such a procedure could be said to come close to 'brain-washing'. Nevertheless, fragrance as a sales device seems to be on the increase. This is evident from the escalation of so-called 'aromatherapy' or 'mood-altering' products on the market today – even if the product in question is a toilet soap scented with synthetics! As for the future:

> It is probable that by the year 2000, managers will use perfumes in department stores the world over as commonly as the US housewives of today use them in their bathrooms, because odorants are potentially more efficacious than any other modality in increasing saleability.[34]

References

1. Stoddart, M., *The Scented Ape*, Cambridge University Press, 1990, p.160.
2. Cited in Weintraub, P., 'Sentimental Journeys' in *Omni*, p.52.
3. Fischer-Rizzi, S., *Complete Aromatherapy Handbook*, Sterling, 1990, p.27.
4. Sugano, H., 'Psychophysiological Studies of Fragrances' in Dodd, G. H. and Van Toller, S., *Fragrance: The Psychology and Biology of Perfume II*, Elsevier Science Publications Ltd., 1992, p.5.
5. Cited in Carrington, H., *Perfumes: Their Sensual Lure and Charm*, Haldeman-Julius Publications, 1947, p.5.
6. Morris, E. T., *Fragrance: The Story of Perfume from Cleopatra to Chanel*, Charles Scribner's Sons, New York, p.47.
7. Tisserand, R., 'Essential Oils as Therapeutic Agents' in Dodd, G. H. and Van Toller, S., *Perfumery: The Psychology and Biology of Fragrance I*, Chapman and Hall, 1990, p.169.
8. Ibid.
9. Steele, J., 'Brain Research and Essential Oils' in *Aromatherapy Quarterly*, Spring 1984.
10. Gattefossé, R. M., *Gattefossé's Aromatherapy*, 1937, reprinted by C. W. Daniel, 1993, p.70.
11. Ibid., p.69.

12. Lorig, T. S., 'Cognitive and non-cognitive effects of odour exposure: electrophysical and behavioural evidence' in Dodd and Van Toller, *Fragrance II*, op. cit., p.162.
13. *International Journal of Aromatherapy*, vol.5, no.2, p.14.
14. Van Toller, *Emotion and the Brain*, 1986, cited in Stoddart, op. cit., p.135.
15. Steele, J. 'Reflections of an Aromatic Archaeologist' in *International Journal of Aromatherapy*, vol.2, no.4, p.8.
16. Ehrlichman, H. and Bastone, L., 'The Use of Odour in the Study of Emotion' in Dodd and Van Toller, *Fragrance II*, op. cit., p.143.
17. Ibid., p.144.
18. Miller, R. A. and I., *The Magical and Ritual Use of Perfumes*, Destiny Books, 1990, p.4.
19. Kirk-Smith, Dr M., 'Human Olfactory Communication', Aroma '93 Conference at Sussex University.
20. King, J. R., 'Anxiety Reduction Using Fragrances' in Dodd and Van Toller, *Perfumery I*, op. cit., p.157.
21. Cited in Weintraub, op. cit., p.52.
22. Schwartz, in *Omni*, p.116.
23. Tagore, R., 'The First Jasmines' from *The Crescent Moon*, Macmillan, 1913, p.71.
24. Cited in King, op. cit., p.154.
25. Drs Warren and Warrenburg, 'The Mood Benefits of Fragrance' in *The International Journal of Aromatherapy*, vol.5, no.2, p.13.
26. Ehrlichman and Bastone, op. cit., p.150.
27. Süskind, P., *Perfume: The Story of a Murderer*, Hamish Hamilton, London, 1986, p.86.
28. Ibid., p.164.
29. McKenzie, D., *Aromatics and the Soul*, Heinemann, 1923, p.44.
30. Dodd and Van Toller, *Perfumery I*, op. cit., p.144.
31. Ehrlichman and Bastone, op. cit., p.143.
32. Dodd and Van Toller, *Perfumery I*, op. cit., p.156.
33. Hirsch, A. R., 'Sensory Marketing' in *The International Journal of Aromatherapy*, vol.5, no.1, p.23.
34. Ibid.

six

The 'Individual Prescription'

> This scent had a freshness, but not the freshness of limes or pomegranates, nor the freshness of myrrh or cinnamon bark or curly mint or birch or camphor or pine needles, nor that of a May rain or a frosty wind or of well water ... and at the same time it had warmth, but not as bergamot, cypress or musk has, or jasmine or narcissi, not as rosewood has or oris ... This scent was inconceivable, indescribable, could not be categorized in any way – it really ought not to exist at all.
>
> Süskind, *Perfume: The Story of a Murderer*, p.42.

In the novel *Perfume*, Grenouille tries unsuccessfully to describe the individual scent of the young woman with whom he is intoxicated, a fragrance so inconceivable that he is possessed by it. Trying to verbalize the 'essence' of a person by their fragrance is a difficult task, especially because, in English at least, there are very few words which may be used to differentiate the nuances of various odours. Nor are we generally aware of the odours of different people or the implications of their specific smell, like Grenouille ... or like a dog. However, in *The Man Who Mistook His Wife For a Hat and Other Clinical Tales* (1985) the neurologist Oliver Sachs recounts an unusual case which gives great insight into what such an experience may be like ...

According to this account, a young medical student of 22 found himself experiencing an enhanced sense of smell for a period of three weeks, after dreaming that he was a bloodhound. He described the experience as evoking 'a strange nostalgia, as of a lost world, half-forgotten, half-recalled', during which he found his sense of smell far more meaningful and personal than his other senses. He discovered that everyone he passed on the street had a distinct 'smell face' which was far more vivid than their 'sight face'. In fact during the whole period of his transformation, he found that his keen olfactory ability told him all he needed to know about the world, for everything was clearly identifiable by its scent – so much so, that his cognitive and intellectual abilities were made redundant!

In the end, our sense of smell is a highly individual phenomenon: it is one way of defining our very personal reality. The scent of a certain perfume or plant may give us a rush and remind us of a childhood sweetheart or it may remind us of a teacher at school whom we hated, it all depends on the context ...

THE IDIOSYNCRATIC NATURE OF SMELL

> In fragrance, there are no absolutes.[1]

There is no doubt that although some fragrances are generally experienced as pleasing and others are perceived as repugnant, it is difficult to make hard and fast rules about how an individual will react to a particular smell. This is because the physiological effect of a given odour can be overridden by specific emotional associations and psychological preferences. Sometimes even an unpleasant smell can have beneficial results if the associations are positive.

Babies can identify and are drawn towards certain odours shortly after birth, for example the scent of their mother's milk. They will also orient towards the scent of the mother's perfume if it has been worn whilst feeding, as opposed to another perfume. According to the child psychiatrist H. J. Schmidt, some odour preferences appear to be innate or acquired very early in infancy, whereas others do not elicit a hedonic response until the child is often over three years old. These two types of reaction to odours are known as a 'hard-wired' response or a 'soft-wired' response: the first is ingrained from before birth and is purely instinctual; the second is learned or acquired later on. So even in young children, it is impossible to predict the response to a certain odour knowing only the nature of the stimulus:

> One must know the age and experimental factors affecting the child's acquisition of the meaning and description of odours. The odour *per se* has no intrinsic effect, although other attributes of the stimulus might.[2]

Thus, in view of the idiosyncratic quality of smell, it is virtually impossible to assess accurately an individual's reaction to a particular odour or to prescribe a particular fragrance for therapeutic purposes without taking all the following considerations into account:

1) *Biological*: what effect the odour is likely to have physiologically on the systems of the body, whether it is stimulating or sedating, etc.

2) *Archetypal*: what universal associations the odour has – the scent of the rose, for example, suggests femininity, love, divinity and sweetness in all cultures alike.

3) *Cultural*: certain scents take on a specific meaning according to the environmental, social and cultural factors involved – the odour of frankincense, for example, will be especially significant to a Roman Catholic.

4) *Individual*: personal associations and preferences due to first-hand experience, which may be either positive or negative.

The need to choose a fragrance specifically tailored or suited to the requirements of each individual, so as to attain the most effective therapeutic results, was the conclusion reached by Marguerite Maury in her work *The Secret of Life and Youth* (1961). She was especially fascinated by the psychological effects of essential oils, and the way in which specific oils could be combined or blended to enhance the personality of her clients, compensate for their imbalances and increase their overall vitality and zest for life:

> But of the greatest interest is the effect of fragrance on the psychic and mental state of the individual. Powers of perception become clearer and more acute and there is a feeling of having, to certain extent, outstripped events. They are seen more objectively, and therefore in truer perspective.[3]

Her attitudes regarding the clarifying properties of fragrance echo those of the great Arab physician Avicenna, who believed that the benefit of 'excellent odours' was that they fortified the senses – 'and when the senses are strong, the thoughts are strong and the conclusions upright'. Eventually, Marguerite Maury devised what she called the 'Individual Prescription' or 'I.P.', a remedy which perfectly mirrored the very identity of each patient, being based on an assessment of their physical, mental and emotional disposition:

> We must, therefore seek odoriferous substances which present affinities with the human being we intend to treat, those which will compensate for his deficiencies and those which will make his faculties blossom. It was by searching for this remedy that we encountered the *individual prescription* (I.P.), which on all points represents the identity of the individual.[4]

The Principles of Perfumery

> Summer's distillation left a prisoner pent in walls of glass.[5]

Before setting out to make a personalized aromatic remedy, it may be useful to keep in mind some of the basic principles of perfumery as it has evolved over the centuries. Perfumery is both a science and an art – it requires precision and sensitivity, but above all the ability to translate an intangible experience or idea into a tangible composition:

> We all possess an imaginary olfactive – a group of olfactive images, often personalized, sometimes in common with others, that the memory has put aside and reconstitutes and compares as soon as we smell a perfume. . . This imaginary olfactive museum is made up of our experiences: the odours of cities, of houses, of men, of women, of a whole book of memories, odours of perfumes, attractive odours, disagreeable odours ... but also, indirectly, of information given to us orally or found in books ... The art of the perfume composer is his capacity to choose and compose using his memories, his passions and his beliefs: and to write the words that will then become perfume.[6]

People generally prefer many-layered fragrance since a combination of different essential oils tends to be more attractive than the smell of a single oil. In addition, the more interesting a perfume smells, the greater its chances for psychological impact. Combining different essential oils makes it possible to totally individualize a blend which is tailored to particular needs. When individual oils are used in combination, the chemical reaction breaks up their original molecular structure and they recombine to form entirely new molecules. The aim is to make a 'bouquet' or a 'seamless scent', where the whole adds up to more than just a sum of its parts. The famous French perfumer Pierre Dhumez spoke of blending perfumes in the following way:

> To make a perfume is to find a harmony of three or four dominant 'bodies' that you smell in your mind. You have an inspiration for a mixture of those three or four bodies, not more. And they will release themselves in such a way that … you will not be able to distinguish one odor from the other among your basic raw materials. It is a perfectly balanced mixture which smells as a separate entity from the odor of each of the three or bodies you have chosen – and in doing so, you have created the 'woman'. After that you have to enhance her – make her more beautiful … and that is a perfume.[7]

Odour direction

Resins				
Wood			OAKMOSS	
Floral		LAVENDER		
Citrus	LIME			
	Top	Middle	Base	***Notes***

The only difference in creating a personalized perfume as opposed to a mass-produced one, is that the 'woman' (or the 'man') is a real person, not simply a figment of the imagination or a fantasy image – like those based on famous personalities such as Coco Chanel or Paloma Picasso.

In composing a perfume, there should also be a balance between the top, middle and base notes. The top notes are the most volatile ingredients; they have a light fresh quality which is immediately apparent – typical top notes include lime, lemon and bergamot. The middle notes constitute the heart of the fragrance and usually form the bulk of the blend – typical middle notes are florals such as lavender, rose or geranium. The base notes gives the fragrance depth and act as fixatives for the more volatile components – typical base notes include oakmoss, benzoin or patchouli.

Although there are over 5,000 natural or synthetic materials available to the modern perfumer, 600 of these comprise the basic ingredients used and only 50 of these basic odours make up 80 per cent of the volume used annually. Thus, although the final touches to a perfume are vital to its overall composition and harmony, they are minimal in terms of amounts used. Some modern commercial perfumes contain well over 100 different ingredients or compounds, but for the purpose of aromatherapy, it is enough to blend between three and seven oils to produce an interesting result.

The birth of perfumery as we know it today occurred as late as the fourteenth century in the West with the discovery of alcoholic extraction techniques. Before that time, perfumes had been based on fatty or oily materials which did not allow the finesse afforded by alcohol. According to Piesse, for example, the original frangipani was composed of every known spice in equal proportions, together with orris powder and one per cent of musk and civet. A liquid scent of the same name was later developed by the inventor's grandson, Mercutio Frangipani, by digesting the powder in alcohol. The result was considered the most lasting of all perfumes made. In more recent years, the name 'frangipani' has been adopted by several different perfume houses as a name for one of their own formulations. It was also incidentally, the name given by French colonists in the West Indies to a species of the genus *Plumieria*.

There are four main principles which characterize odour perception, namely quality, intensity, duration and volatility. Such factors depend on how a perfume has been constructed. Modern commercial perfumes vary in strength, depending upon the ratio of essence to alcohol. *Parfum* (up to 30 per cent essence) is the strongest; then *Eau de parfum* (10–15 per cent); then *Eau de toilette* (5–10 per cent); followed by *Cologne* (2–6 per cent). Individual skin characteristics and odour play a role in how a perfume will react with body chemistry. Oily skin absorbs and retains odour molecules more easily than dry skin; those with dry skin should therefore use a more concentrated type of fragrance. Some people prefer to wear a single signature scent, while others have several perfumes to suit different moods.

For aromatherapy purposes, it is recommended that the chosen essential oils are blended with a base oil such as jojoba or fractionated coconut in a 50–50 ratio as opposed to dissolving them in an alcoholic base. The essential oils should be added slowly, pausing at every stage, starting with the middle notes, then the base notes and finally the top notes. Such a blend will take about a month to 'mature' fully. This gives a concentrated 'unguent' style scent, which is very long lasting. Moreover, in aromatherapy, it is possible to blend an individual perfume which is composed of wholly natural ingredients (as all perfumes once were), rather than one containing synthetics, like most modern perfumes.

Personalized Perfumes

> In Paris, in the time of our great grandparents, the 'Golden Age of Perfumery' still lived on. Our great grandmothers would consult with their perfumer. He would make, exclusively for them, a special perfume. The formula was a secret and our great grandmothers would never tell anyone what their delightful perfume was, so much was it part of their personality.[8]

The idea of matching a perfume to the personality of its wearer is not a new idea. An English physician of the last century had stated that, in his opinion, each perfume should correspond to the physical, emotional and mental characteristics of its wearer, and proceeded to ask:

> Why should we not know our fair friends by the delicate odours with which they are surrounded, as we know them far off by the sound of their voice? The *spirituelle* should affect jasmine; the *brilliante* and witty magnolia; the robust the more musky odours; and young girls, just blooming into womanhood, the rose. The citron-like perfumes are more suited to the melancholy temperament, and there is a sad note in heliotrope that the young widow should affect.[9]

Several centuries earlier, Theophrastus had considered that the perfumes 'Egyptian' and 'Megalleion' were best suited to women, being 'heavy' and long-lasting, whereas men were better sprinkling the lighter, powdered 'Susinum' on their beds. Gradually, various theories developed regarding the suitability of certain perfumes to individual people based on sex, nationality, age, hair colouring, personality type, disposition, etc.

> For a perfume to fulfil its function to the maximum extent it is important that it is tailored to the wearer's natural odour signature ... The key to the structure of a personal perfume is hair colour which is, as is well known, closely related to skin colour.[10]

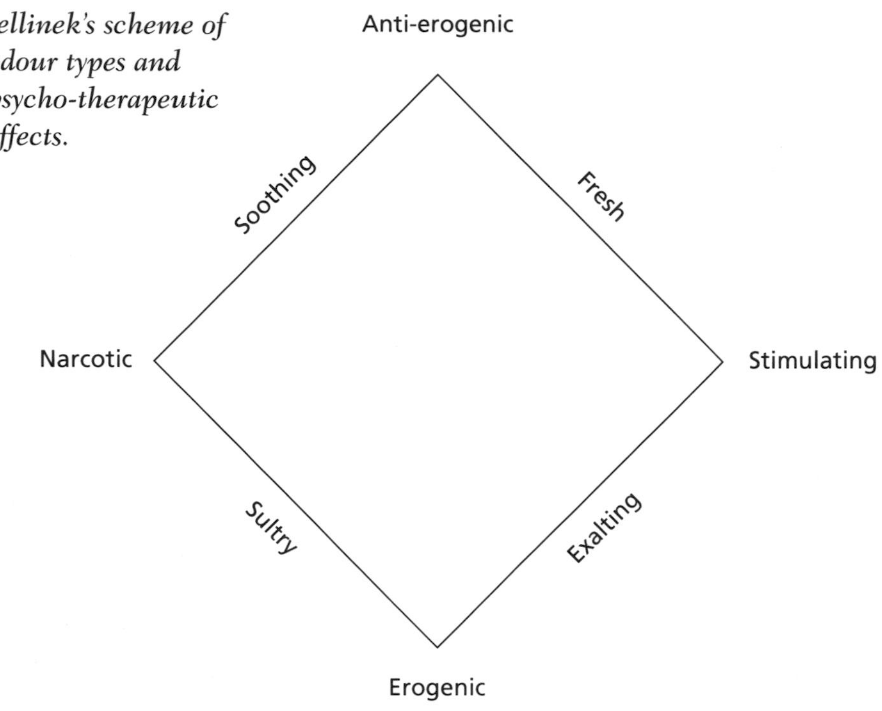

Jellinek's scheme of odour types and psycho-therapeutic effects.

People of different race are suited to different types of perfume and tend to display distinct preferences: Western Europeans favour subtle, sophisticated fragrances; natives of African and the Middle East prefer heavier, spicy, more sultry aromas; Americans tend to like strong, vital perfumes; while the Scandinavians gravitate towards light, refreshing scents. On this basis, the Austrian perfumer Jellinek (1954) classified perfumes primarily according to hair colouring:

Blonde – *fresh; stimulating and not strongly erogenic*
Black – *sultry; erogenic and intoxicating (narcotic)*
Brunette – *soothing; intoxicating and not strongly erogenic*
Red – *exalting; erogenic and stimulating*

A reddish-blonde type will harmonize with a stimulating perfume, a dark brunette type with a narcotic perfume. Any disharmonies which also become evident from the diagram are felt even stronger in practice than the harmonies. Such disharmonies exist between the black type and fresh odours ... blonde hair and 'sultry' perfumes, such as Oriental perfumes etc.11

More subtle, however, are the notions based on personality types, where the emphasis is on finding a psychological correspondence between the 'essence' of a person and the 'essence' of a perfume. This idea, which has much in common with M. Maury's own concepts, has gained increasing respect recently:

> The correlation between personality and fragrance was initially a supposition, but the latest research in the psycho-physiological area supports this idea.[12]

R. W. Moncrieff was one of the first to correlate different scents with different types of people. He noted that extroverts were less finely tuned in their odour preferences than introverts, and they tended to prefer lighter fragrances, while introverts tended to favour the heavier, oriental scents. Mensing and Beck developed these notions a great deal further, using what they called the colour rosette test.[13] This consisted of a panel of eight circles, each with eight different overlapping colour segments. The colours within each circle were carefully chosen to match the preferences of the eight most common personality types, that is:

1) Orange/yellow/red/green: 'extroverted mood tendency' – readiness to take risks, sociable, likes stimulation: fresh (green) notes.

2) Purple/violet/white: 'introverted mood tendency' – needs inner tranquillity, less need for stimulation, individual/alternative life-style, younger age group: oriental notes.

3) Black and white: 'emotionally ambivalent mood tendency' – highly sensitive, 'moody', romantic, fashion-oriented: floral powdery notes.

4) Bright colours (yellow/pink/red/blue/orange) – 'emotionally ambivalent with extroverted mood tendency' – idealistic, cheerful, impulsive, satisfied and content with life, young and old age group: floral fruity notes.

5) Dark green/violet/warm colours: 'emotionally ambivalent with introverted mood tendency' – materialistic, needs security, avoids conflicts, likes a feeling of stability: oriental floral notes.

6) Dark red/green/orange: 'emotionally stable with extroverted mood tendency' – conservative, socially active, family oriented, radiates warmth and strength, likes good quality, well-made things: chypre notes.

7) Blue/yellow/silver grey: 'emotionally stable with introverted mood tendency' – well-mannered, self-controlled, does not overstep others' boundaries, likes things elegant and precious: aldehydic floral notes.

8) Brown/green/yellow: 'indefinable' – straightforward, uncomplicated: people with very stable moods do not have a typical preferred fragrance.

The colour scheme to which an individual was attracted gave an immediate insight into their personality type and thus their odour preferences. This is because our response to colour is dealt with in the limbic system, the same part of the brain which registers smells. Different colours, like different scents, tend to evoke particular feelings and the way we interact with the world is expressed through our emotional relationships with it. In general, extroverts tend to be attracted to fresh scents because they enjoy more stimulation, whereas introverts prefer oriental perfumes because they are generally more reflective. Those with changeable moods are drawn to floral fragrances, while those with the most balanced emotions, curiously, show no odour preferences.

Although the colour chart has only been utilized in the realm of perfumery, similar notions can be applied in psycho-aromatherapy in helping to correlate specific essential oils with different personality types. An introverted individual, for example, is more likely to be attracted to oriental oils and incense materials, such as frankincense, patchouli, sandalwood or galbanum, while an extroverted type will tend to prefer a predominance of fresh or citrus oils such as myrtle, bergamot, lemon or grapefruit.

But when we move into the therapeutic use of essences, techniques such as the colour rosette test lose their effectiveness, for there are other factors to be considered:

> While the perfume exists by and for itself, as self-sufficient, and represents an end in itself, the I.P., identical with the individual for whom it has been

concocted, is in intimate relationship with the latter ... Almost invariably the odour, and above all the fragrance of the I.P., express and almost depict the person, feature by feature. Gay or sad, charmer or sour. The impression [and] the sensation suggested by the perfume are exactly the same as those felt on contact with the person.[14]

In perfumery, the aesthetic consideration is paramount, while in therapeutic work, the efficacy of the remedy is of prime importance. In addition, when dealing with the therapeutic application of essences, there are two interrelated dynamics to take into consideration:

1) The *signature scent* – i.e. the fragrance which corresponds to the physical, emotional and mental characteristics of the wearer.

2) The *regulating agents* – i.e. ingredients which are needed to balance what is absent in the health or personality of the wearer.

It is for this reason that Madame Maury likened the I.P. to 'the negative of a film with its reversed shadows and light',[15] which when 'developed', portrayed the 'true' form of the person. For, as the patient changed, so the mixture changed too – one or several of the essences would have to be eliminated and replaced by another as the treatment progressed.

Creative blending is an aesthetic alchemical process ... learning to 'listen through the nose'. To listen is to be receptive, to be empty. Every drop shifts the orchestration of olfactory vibrations, the 'song of the blend'. A blend is not made at once, rather it evolves, it organically grows and interacts not only with the essential oils, but also with the blender.[16]

Hippocrate's Four Humours/Temperaments

Element	*Humour*	*Season*	*Temperature*	*Moisture*
Air	Sanguine	Spring	Hot	Wet
Fire	Choleric	Summer	Hot	Dry
Earth	Melancholic	Autumn	Cold	Dry
Water	Phlegmatic	Winter	Cold	Wet

The Remedial Power of Opposites

The remedial power of opposites is based on an ancient concept, including the four element and four humour theory of Hippocrates:
In his *Classification and Description of the Temperaments*, the eighteenth-century physician Gaub wrote:

- In that called the sanguine temperament, an easily taught, ready, generous and flexible disposition is coupled with negligence, want of foresight, inconstancy, immoderacy and an unbridled love of pleasure.

- You will praise the pungent spirit and glowing imagination, the fiery readiness for action and the steadfastness of the choleric man, but you will deplore the ready rashness to dare all, and the harsh irascibility and

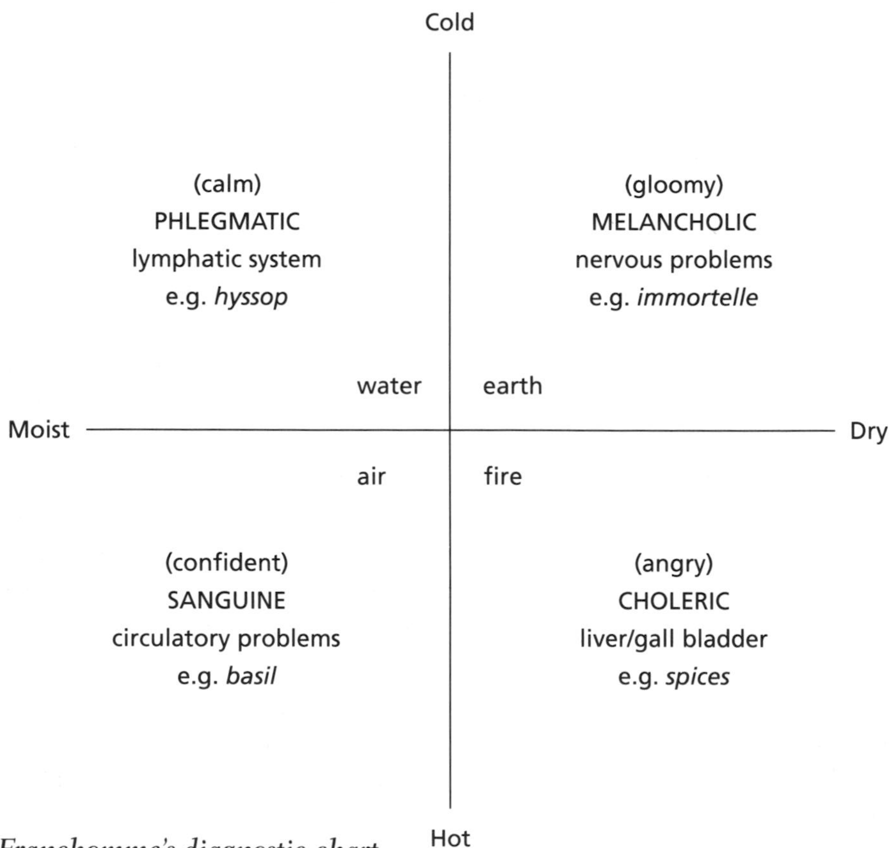

Franchomme's diagnostic chart.

insufferable pride with which they are coupled.

• In the melancholic constitution everything is the opposite. The understanding is slow but most penetrating, the power of attention is tireless and pursuit of whatever has been initiated is tenacious. They are prudent beyond measure, covetous and suspicious, and their emotions are sluggish indeed but hard to suppress.

• Finally, shall I arouse the sleepy phlegmatics, unresponsive to everything, striving greatly for nothing, of whom it may be said that they live for their gullets and bellies alone.[17]

Air opposes Earth, Fire opposes Water ... therefore according to this theory, remedies for a watery or phlegmatic type of person or disease would be found among the fiery remedies such as cinnamon, cassia or cardamom, which are all 'warming and drying'. This method of diagnosis was very popular in the practice of herbal medicine throughout the eighteenth century, but is equally applicable to the realm of aromatics today (see also Appendix III: Astrological Correspondences).

The four humour theory has been applied to aromatherapy by Dr Pierre Franchomme. He uses it to help understand and deal with the basic temperament of his patients. For example, he recommends that a melancholic type of person should have hot baths which are both relaxing and re-energizing, using essential oils of the moist/hot type, such as basil. If a person is very depressed it means they are losing vital energy and are in need of heat and energy to revitalize the system. On the other hand, a sanguine type of person, who is more likely to suffer from heart problems and high blood pressure, is in need of soothing and cooling treatments using an oil such as immortelle. Bilious, liverish-type people should be treated with oils containing principally *esters* and *ketones*. Yet, since most aromatics fit into the 'hot and dry' category, it would seem to suggest that it is the sanguine, sleepy type of person who can benefit most from the regular use of aromatic oils, such as angelica, aniseed, cinnamon, clove, frankincense, ginger, juniper, cypress and pine!

In *Essential Oils as Psychotherapeutic Agents*, Robert Tisserand proposes eight mood categories which may be used to chart 'our personal mood cycle' where certain essential oils are used to help counteract or balance extremes of emotion:

> Positive turns to negative when our mood takes over and starts to control us to an unwelcome degree. When this happens, one solution may be aromatherapy. The appropriate essential oil forms a counter-vibration to that of the negative mood, so restoring harmony ... [18]

Here, the essential oils are described in terms of the mood which they generally evoke, although these are subject to individual experience. Ylang ylang, for example, because it inspires passion, can help combat

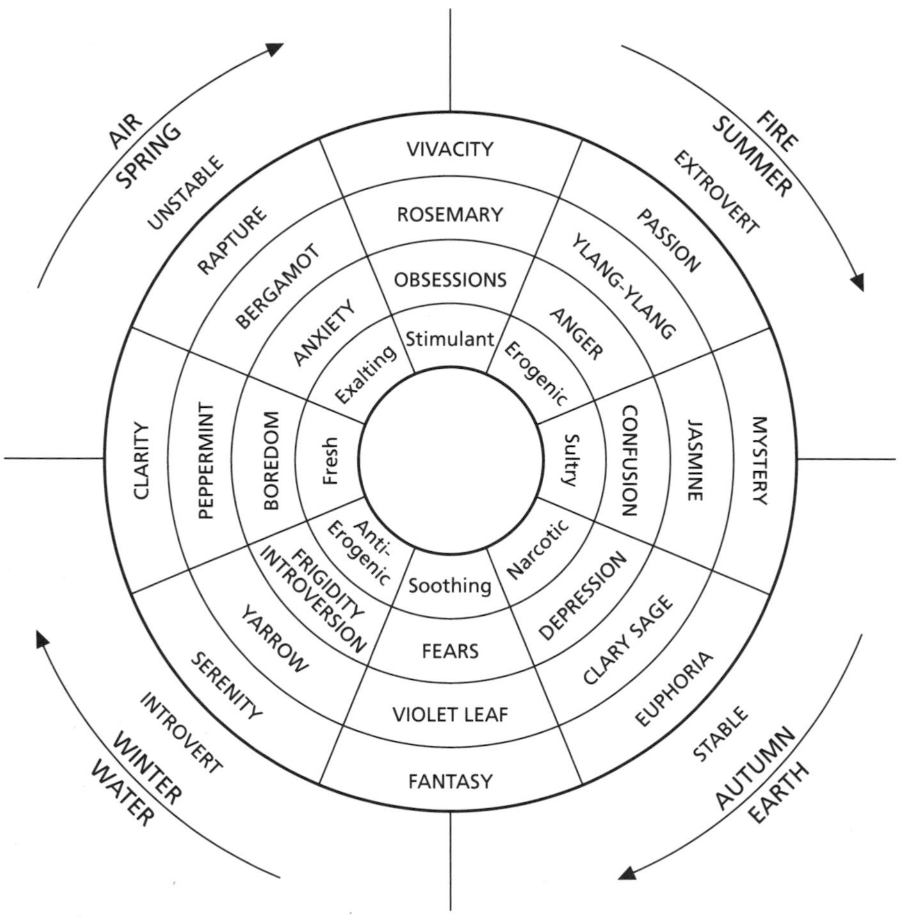

The mood cycle, showing correspondences with the four elements and typical essential oils.

frigidity and introversion. Jasmine, which is often worn as a perfume in its own right due to its intriguing, sultry fragrance, may also be a valuable addition to the I.P. of a person who is uninspired, bored and in need of new ideas. The dangers of such a scheme, however, lie in the limitations which it tends to impose; in addition, there is a danger in defining the emotional effects of essential oils in too much detail, because of differing personal temperaments and individual associations.

In assessing the needs of an individual, aesthetic preferences often correspond to suitability and can be of great value as a therapeutic guide. Much as our body may at times crave certain foods which can supply the type of nutrition or vitamins which are lacking, so may we be emotionally drawn towards particular fragrances that have a balancing effect on our psychic disposition as a whole. As Christine Wildwood says:

> Time and time again it has been observed that we are instinctively drawn to the essential oil that is right for our needs at the time and, as our emotional state alters, so might our aroma preference.[19]

This involves trusting the intuition and the feelings. And since it has been found that pleasing scents have greater access to the brain and central nervous system than those experienced as repulsive or indifferent, the therapeutic potential of a favourite aroma is also greater.

In reality, most people are drawn to a number of different scents or oils simultaneously – for each evokes a positive, pleasurable effect in its own way. Sometimes one particular oil may stand out as having an almost addictive quality to it, while the others have a somewhat lesser or even surprising attraction. Whatever the case, a person's choice will often indicate a preference for a certain group of oils. For example, someone may favour light, fresh, floral scents, while at the same time displaying an antipathy towards another class, such as those with a heavy, musky, resinous aroma. Often, a person's aroma preferences can demonstrate a good deal about their disposition – whether they need to be stimulated or soothed and what psychological factors are at work.

In conclusion, there is no doubt that on a personal level, essential oils can help to bring about a change in the health of an individual. By supporting their strengths and countering their weaknesses, natural aromatic remedies can help balance emotional disturbances and restore the original harmony and unity of the personality, especially when they are tailored to the individual's specific personality and needs.

But what about the underlying causes? Pollution, stress, social and environmental problems all contribute to the negative attitudes, moods and feelings which in turn deplete the immune system and eventually lead to disease. So many modern complaints are due to conditions outside the individual's control, resulting in feelings of hopelessness and despair. Since our emotional state has a direct influence on the ability of a virus to enter the cells of the body, using essential oils to cultivate a positive mental attitude can do much to prevent the onset of disease at its roots.

At the Aroma '93 Conference, 'Harmony from Within', Dr Kurt Schnaubelt emphasized the importance of emotional factors in helping to prevent and combat 'civilisation diseases', and the ability of oils such as clove, cinnamon and citrus oils to alleviate headaches, lift the spirits, improve self-esteem and encourage feelings of well-being. These qualities should not be underestimated! According to Dr Daniel Pénöel:

> Aromatic medicine is a preventative healing focusing on the evolutionary side of all living beings of the Biosphere, be it in the vegetable or animal kingdom. Aromatic medicine ... could eventually become the ecological medicine of the 21st century by balancing earth, water and atmospheric ecosystems.[20]

Seen in this context, essential oils provide the ideal components of *preventative* medicine: they not only support the immune system and help to prevent illness because of their physiological properties – bactericidal, fungicidal, prophylactic, antiseptic etc. – but also they can exert a positive psychological effect, a factor which is increasingly being explored in the field of environmental fragrancing.

New Directions

> The science of aromatherapy ... promises to revolutionize the workplace and the home. In the not-too-distant future, office ventilation systems might emit aromas that stimulate workers yet help them to relax. Scent machines as elaborate as stereo systems might churn vapours through the home, acting as aphrodisiacs and alarm clocks. And for those on the road a scratch card ... might provide an array of odours to fit conditions from anxiety and claustrophobia to migraine.[21]

Essential oils are already being used increasingly in public places to enhance the immediate environment – notably in the USA and Japan. At the Plane Tree Hospital in California, (where the patient is placed at the centre of his or her own treatment), patients are given a choice of sensory modalities including a choice of fragrance. At the St Croix Valley Memorial Hospital, Wisconsin, natural fragrances are used to counteract unpleasant odours and improve the atmosphere of the main lobby, the chemical dependence room and the nurses' office. In New York City's Sloane-Kettering Institute, which is devoted to cancer research, clinical tests demonstrated that *heliotropin*, a vanilla-like scent, reduced anxiety. Recent studies have also shown that peppermint and lily-of-the-valley eased depression and improved self-esteem.

In the United Kingdom, some hospitals regularly vaporize oils such as lavender or chamomile in the wards to lift anxiety and increase a feeling of well-being among patients. At the Old Manor Hospital in Salisbury, Mark Hardy, RMN, conducted an experiment to assess the effects of lavender oil on the sleeping patterns of elderly mentally ill patients, in place of their usual medication. In these initial tests, he used a vortex air freshener to vaporize the lavender oil into the ward at night, with the following results:

> Residents exhibited less restlessness during the night, their sleep was deeper and so they were not being woken while staff made their rounds, there were fewer periods of simple insomnia and the mood of residents on waking was more pleasant ... There was even a slight increase in the hours of sleep obtained using lavender oil as opposed to night medication.[22]

In addition:

> The dormitory's environment was improved for everyone, as the oil masked the unpleasant odours that can occur in an elderly ward. It left the atmosphere fresh and lightly perfumed.[23]

At the St Nicholas Therapy Unit in Shoreham, Sussex, a blend of chamomile, ylang ylang and lavender has been employed in foot massage treatments to help 'calm and relax or stimulate and uplift the clients'. With repeated massage treatments, patients with mental disabilities and communication problems gradually became more relaxed and less anxious and for those with profound handicaps, aromatherapy was found to be 'invaluable as a means of making them feel involved and cared for'.[24]

Neroli oil has also been used in foot massage treatments in the intensive care unit of Middlesex Hospital with positive results, especially with regard to its relaxing, soothing qualities. It was also found to produce a marked reduction in anxiety among patients.[25]

Japan has also shown a keen interest in utilizing aromatic oils within the hospital environment. According to Sugano of the Japan School of Medicine, natural fragrances can provide a cost-effective and efficient alternative to many common drug treatments, especially the use of stimulants and tranquillizers which often have addictive, toxic and other side-effects. He believes that 'aromatherapy' is still in its infancy and that:

> Increasingly, we can expect to find the use of fragrances in hospitals to help in the relaxation of patients as well as in the workplace to help increase the work output.[26]

In Japan, the Shimuzu Construction Corporation of Tokyo has already developed a computerized scent-delivery system. Originally made to combat the effects of interior air pollution, the system first filters and purifies the air and then scents it as it is circulated. In 1985, the Japanese began testing the effects of natural plant oils on employees' cognitive brain processes in the work environment. They found that by utilizing cephalic oils like lemon or grapefruit, their office staff benefited from reduced illness, increased feelings of job satisfaction and higher standards of achievement. In addition, R. Baron[27] found that people working in the presence of a pleasant odour set higher goals and were more likely to employ an efficient strategy than subjects working in an unscented room.

The Japanese also found that the amount of concentrated essence required to have a tangible effect was actually very low and that the most advantageous point of awareness occurred when the level of fragrance was above the conscious threshold, but not obtrusive – in other words, it remained in the background. Also important was the 'wafting effect', for if any fragrance was used at the same level and same concentration over a period of time, the effect of the scent was dulled. However, whether an individual was conscious of the fragrance or not, it was observed that the effect on the mind continued, since the aromatic molecules were still 'dynamic within the biochemistry of the nervous system'.[28]

Shops and hotels are also beginning to experiment with the effects of different odours on the psychological disposition of their customers. The Miami Marriott Hotel in the USA has recently installed a fragrance generator that releases a unique floral/citrus blend into the lobby through the central air-conditioning system. The fragrance, called 'Mango', was specially formulated by aromatic consultant John Steele and made entirely from natural plant extracts. 'The desired effect is to alleviate stress,' says Richard Dodd, and has been especially tailored to the hotel's Central and South American guests who 'lean more towards floral appreciation'.[29] According to Mark Peltier:

> These scents can be customized for each customer's needs, and signature blends can reflect the distinct theme of each property or project … we see the future of environmental fragrancing as a dynamic interaction between the individual and his environment and the opportunity to bring a healthier, refreshing air quality indoors.[30]

Some airlines are also beginning to utilize the properties of pure essential oils to help their customers overcome travel fatigue and jet lag. Virgin Air-lines has recently commissioned Aqua Oleum to formulate three specific blends, called 'Sweet Breezes', which are relaxing, refreshing or comforting in effect, and New Zealand Airlines is already using a special blend of aromas in its planes to ward off airsickness among passengers.

Specially formulated essential oils blends are increasingly being used in the gym (especially in the sauna) and to enhance the atmosphere in exhibition halls. Perhaps in the future, they may even be used in theatres, as they were in Roman times:

> Think how the appeal of a love scene would be strengthened by an invisible cloud of roses blown into the house through the ventilating shaft.[31]

An American company is currently preparing to market an olfactory cassette player, which will allow people to select a scent from a case of odour 'cartridges', while in Japan, a clock maker already sells an alarm clock that arouses the sleeper by scenting the room with a formula to stimulate alertness! The psychologist Susan Schiffman of Duke University has developed such ideas even further – she has found, for example, that a chocolate-scented spray applied to the back of the tongue can help curb desires for the actual thing and that peach scent alleviates pain. Schiffman's notion that hard-wired receptors travel from the nose to specific sites in the brain presages significant breakthroughs in the therapeutic use of odours:

> Once we figure out which substances stimulate which receptors ... and how these substances connect with parts of the brain, we'll be able to design bullets of odor that act like drugs.[32]

Such possibilities hold particular value because of the limitations imposed by the blood-brain barrier – the lipid membrane which covers the capillaries carrying blood past the brain. Up to now, it has been impossible to target such brain maladies as Alzheimer's disease using conventional drugs, because the molecules are too large to penetrate the blood-brain barrier. The olfactory nerves, on the other hand, which evolved *before* the brain, are the only neurons not protected by the sheath. Thus they offer the only natural means of treating the brain directly.

> This seems to be the magic pathway ... Ten years from now, odor pharmacologists will be designing two-part molecules. The first part will be targeted to specific receptors in the nose. The second part will have therapeutic or medicinal effects on targeted areas of the brain.[33]

In short, by the use of fragrance, it will soon be possible to influence the mind directly and treat brain sites 'implicated in disease, emotion and thought'. The olfactory revolution is already underway!

References

1. John Steele.
2. Engen, T., 'The Acquisition of Odour Hedonics' in Dodd, G. H. and Van Toller, S., *Perfumery: The Psychology and Biology of Fragrance I*, Chapman and Hall, 1990. p.60.
3. Maury, M., *Marguerite Maury's Guide to Aromatherapy*, C. W. Daniel, 1989, p.82.
4. Ibid., p.94.
5. Shakespeare, William, 'Fifth Sonnet'.
6. Ellena, J. C., 'Creative Perfumery' in Muller, R. M. and Lamparsky, D., *Perfumes: Art, Science, Technology*, Elsevier Applied Science, 1991, p.342.
7. Cited in Miller, R. A. and I., *The Magical and Ritual Use of Perfumes*, Destiny Books, 1990, p.16.
8. Le Norcy, S., 'Selling Perfume: A Technique or an Art?' in Dodd and Van Toller, *Perfumery I*, op. cit., p.219.
9. Cited in Carrington, H., *Perfumes, Their Sensual Lure and Charm*, Haldeman-Julius Publications, 1947, p.4.
10. Cited in Stoddart, D. M., *The Scented Ape*, Cambridge University Press, 1990, p.164.
11. Ibid., p.165.
12. Mensing and Beck, 'The Psychology of Perfume Selection ' in Dodd and Van Toller, *Perfumery I*, op. cit., p.185.
13. Ibid.
14. Maury, op. cit., p.98.
15. Ibid., p.95.
16. Cited in Lawless, J., *The Encyclopaedia of Essential Oils*, Element Books, 1992, p.33.
17. Cited in Rather, L. J., *Mind and Body in 18th Century Medicine*, Wellcome Historical Medical Library, 1965, p.88.
18. Tisserand, R., 'Essential Oils as Therapeutic Agents' in Dodd, G. H. and Van Toller, S., *Perfumery I*, op. cit., p.179.
19. Wildwood, C., *Creative Aromatherapy*, Thorsons, 1993, p.106.
20. Cited in *Beyond Scents*, Spring 1993, p.8.
21. Weintraub, P., 'Sentimental Journeys' in *Omni*, p.52.
22. Hardy, M., 'Sweet Scented Dreams' in *The International Journal of Aromatherapy*, vol.3, no.1, p.13.
23. Ibid.
24. *The International Journal of Aromatherapy*, vol.2, no.1, p.17.

25. Ibid., vol.4, no.3, p.24.
26. Sugano, H., 'Psychophysical Studies of Fragrances' in Dodd, G. H. and Van Toller, S., *Fragrance: The Psychology and Biology of Perfume II*, Elsevier Science Publications Ltd., 1992, p.227.
27. Baron, R., 'Environmentally induced positive effect' in *The Journal of Applied Social Psychology*, vol.16, 1990, pp.16–28.
28. *Beyond Scents*, Spring 1993, p.7.
29. *The Wall Street Journal*, 28 July, 1992.
30. *Beyond Scents*, op. cit.
31. McKenzie, D., *Aromatics and the Soul*, Heinemann, 1923, p.57.
32. Cited in Weintraub, op. cit., p.116.
33. Ibid.

2

A Guide to Selected Essential Oils

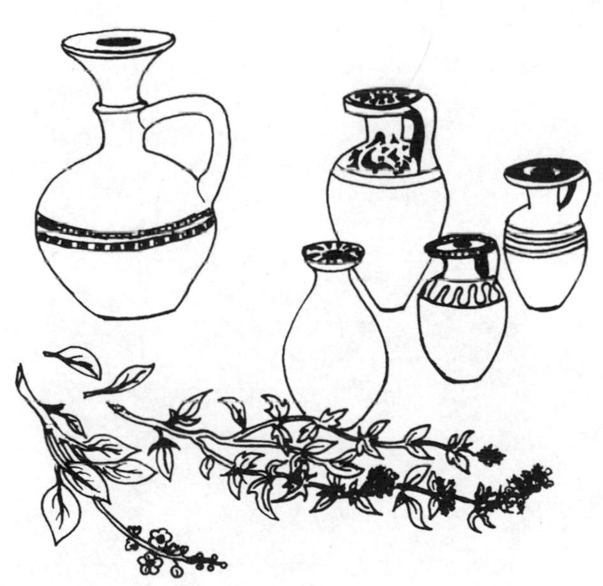

ANGELICA *Angelica archangelica*

Renowned since antiquity, angelica was used to purify the blood, prevent the spread of infection and protect from all kinds of evil. According to a tenth-century French tale, the Archangel Raphael revealed the virtues of this aromatic plant to a monk in a dream, so it might be used as an antidote to the plague.

The whole herb was traditionally associated with the sun and with Venus. Angelica stems were chewed as a preventative and the seeds and roots burned to purify the air. The yellow juice from the roots was an ingredient of 'Carmelite water', a remedy used to promote long life and to protect against 'enchantments, poysons and the spells of wytches';[1] the root was also used as a protective amulet.

In Eastern Prussia and the surrounding regions it was the custom as part of an early pagan celebration for peasants to march into town chanting an ancient ditty and carrying the flowering stems of angelica. Later, because it was seen to flower on the 8 May, St Michael the Archangel's day, it became known as the 'Herb of the Holy Ghost' and associated with the Spring Annunciation festivities.

A type of Virginian angelica was known to the Native Americans as 'Hunting or Fishing Root', because if rubbed on the hands it attracted fish and game. In herbal medicine, especially in China, angelica is still used a great deal to

SCENT:
Balsamic, bitter-sweet, earthy, herbaceous, long-lasting, musky, powerful, spicy. The root oil has a scent like a mixture of pepper and musk; the seed oil is fresher and more spicy.
It blends well with bergamot, clary sage, juniper, lemon, orange, patchouli, pine and vetiver.

KEY QUALITIES:
Comforting, earthy, fiery, fixative, grounding, protective, purifying, restorative, revitalizing, sedating (in large doses), stimulating (in small quantities), warming.

CONTRA-INDICATIONS:
The root oil is phototoxic, i.e. can cause pigmentation on skin exposed to direct sunlight; best avoided during pregnancy and by diabetics.

promote fertility and as a general tonic. The Laplanders chew the root like tobacco to promote long life. In Western herbalism, it is used to strengthen and comfort the heart, as it is good for palpitations and 'exhilarates and revives the melancholic person'.[2]

In aromatherapy, the essential oil is used as a general restorative and stimulant of the nervous system, although it is soporific in excess. It has a strong fiery quality, which is good for all types of nervous debility.

> This essential oil is helpful for those who are afraid, timid, weak, or who lack perseverance and have a tough time making decisions. Angelica aids people with an upset nervous system who urgently need to rebuild body and soul.[3]

APPLICATIONS & METHODS OF USE:

- To strengthen body and mind, add 5–10 drops to the bath. Good for mental fatigue, migraine, headaches, nervous depression and general debility.
- Add a few drops to a vaporizer to make an uplifting, purifying incense for meditation, yoga, etc. – it promotes good respiration and deepens the breath. The vaporized oil also helps prevent the spread of infection and makes a pleasing room fragrance.
- For a massage oil, add 6 drops to 1 Tbs sweet almond oil. It stimulates the circulation and the brain and strengthens the nerves.
- Add the oil or herb to pot pourris, etc.
- To help counteract anxiety, nausea or dizziness, put a few drops on a hanky and inhale throughout the day.

ANISEED *Pimpinella anisum*

Aniseed, the seed of anise, an airy spice under the domination of Jupiter, was believed to keep away nightmares, having an overall purifying and protecting quality; it was also thought to avert the 'evil eye': 'The seeds bound in linnen cloath and smelled unto prevent evil dreams.'[4]

It was cultivated by the ancient Egyptians as a medicine and culinary spice, and was thought to 'refresh the heart'. It was well known to the Greeks and Romans: Pliny recommended taking aniseed with honey and myrrh in the morning as a 'pick-me-up'. The oil was traditionally used for vertigo and to strengthen the nerves.

Anise, combined with orris, was employed by Edward IV for scenting linen and clothes, as recorded in his wardrobe accounts of 1480.

The seeds of the closely related star anise (*Illicium verum*) are used in China to sweeten the breath and in Japan the tree is planted in temples and on graves, while the powdered bark is used as incense. It is also used as a fumigant and as an insect repellent.

SCENT:
Liquorice-like, rich, spicy sweet, very pervasive.
It blends well with lavender, pine, rose and other spicy oils.

KEY QUALITIES:
Aphrodisiac, comforting, protective, purifying, reviving, soothing, stimulant (in small doses), stupefying (in excess), uplifting, warming.

CONTRA-INDICATIONS:
Narcotic in large doses; possible sensitization: use in moderation only. Star anise should not be used in therapy.

In Tibetan medicine a lotion containing aniseed and nutmeg in melted butter is recommended for anxiety, hysteria, depression and other neurotic symptoms. Aniseed is also included in the preparation of 'Aquilaria A', which contains 31 aromatic ingredients, 'and is one of the most potent stress relieving agents particularly when its medicated fumes are inhaled'.[5]

The essential oil acts as a general stimulant in small doses, but is stupefying in excess. The warm spicy scent has an uplifting and comforting effect on the mind. It also has the reputation for having aphrodisiac properties. It is good for introverted, melancholic or fearful people who tend to be withdrawn or frigid.

APPLICATIONS & METHODS OF USE:

- Use up to 5 drops in the bath for nervous headaches, anxiety, stress, insomnia and general exhaustion.
- Use a few drops in a vaporizer as a purifying and reviving room fragrance. It promotes good respiration, clears the head and strengthens the nerves.

- Make a tisane by boiling 2 tsps of seeds in 1 pint (600 ml) of water for 3 minutes. Let it steep and sip slowly with honey as required. Good for nervous indigestion, palpitations and as a general relaxant, also helpful for PMT and menopausal problems.
- For a soothing, comforting massage oil, mix 2 drops each of aniseed, nutmeg and rose with 1 Tbs sweet almond oil.
- The seeds or oil make a good addition to pot pourris.

BASIL *Ocimum basilicum*

Basil has a history of mixed associations – on the one hand its name is thought to derive from the Greek *basileus*, meaning 'royal', and on the other from a mythical lizard-like monster 'basilisk', said to have a fatal glance and breath.

In Crete, basil symbolized 'love washed with tears', and was associated with death and evil. The Greeks believed that the plant should be sown while uttering words of abuse, or it would not flourish.

In contrast, the Romans considered it to be an aphrodisiac and a symbol of strength and in Italy the herb is still used as a love token, worn behind the ear.

In the sixteenth century it was made into a powder and inhaled like snuff, to help relieve headaches or congestion. According to Culpeper it was under the domination of Mars and under Scorpio. It was also used as a strewing herb, due its fine fragrance, and to scent linen and washing water.

The herbalist John Gerard wrote,

> The smell of basil is good for the heart … it taketh away sorrowfulness, which commeth of melancholy, and maketh a man merry and glad.[6]

In India, this plant is held sacred to Krishna and Vishnu – Vishnu's wife Lakshmi was transformed into *tulasi* or holy basil. Its leaves are placed on the breasts of the dead as protection for their soul. It is grown in pots near temples and outside nearly every house, watered daily and worshipped by all members of the household. The root is made into beads and the seeds into rosaries. It is still highly esteemed in Ayurvedic medicine, especially for its anti-infectious properties.

The herb was also known to the ancient Egyptians and wreaths of basil have been found in the burial chambers of the pyramids. In Egypt today, the leaves are scattered on graves.

The Jews hold sprays of basil in their hands during religious fasts to give them strength.

SCENT:
Clove-like, fresh, slightly spicy.
It blends well with citrus oils, especially bergamot or orange, geranium and other herbal aromas such as clary sage or rosemary.

KEY QUALITIES:
Clearing, fiery, fortifying, insect repellent, purifying, refreshing, restorative, strengthening, stimulant (adrenal cortex), tonic, uplifting, warming.

CONTRA-INDICATIONS:
Stupefying in excess: use in moderation only. Some types of basil may cause sensitization of the skin. Use only a few drops in the bath, otherwise it causes a tingling sensation.

There are many varieties of basil used to produce essential oils, each containing a distinct blend of constituents and having different aromatic qualities, the most common types being the 'exotic' and 'sweet' basil. The sweet basil is safer for therapeutic purposes, having a fresh, penetrating, sweet herbaceous aroma. The fragrance alone strengthens the nerves, stimulates the adrenal cortex, clears the head and gives the mind strength and clarity.

In aromatherapy, it is used as a restorative and general nerve tonic. It has a reviving, refreshing effect on the mind and spirits. This oil is good for those in need of protection, due either to a debilitating illness and low resistance levels, nervous exhaustion, a constitutional weakness or a change in life resulting in feelings of vulnerability. It is helpful for intellectual fatigue, for exams and during long periods of study.

APPLICATIONS & METHODS OF USE:

- Use up to 5 drops in a morning bath for all types of debility – nervous headaches, anxiety, migraine, stress-related complaints, listlessness, depression, nervous exhaustion, mental fatigue and poor memory.
- Put a few drops on a hanky for use throughout the day for morning sickness, travel sickness, dizziness, exam nerves and nausea. It can also help restore loss of smell due to congestion.
- Basil is a useful oil to vaporize in a room to prevent the spread of infection and to get rid of unwanted smells, such as cigarette smoke. The few drops of oil in a vaporizer may also be used to keep flies and mosquitoes away.
  A sprig of basil in the wardrobe keeps moths away.
- Best blended with other oils for massage, e.g. 2 drops each of clary sage, bergamot and basil in 1 Tbs sweet almond oil.
- Used as an incense, the scent is conducive to meditation, yoga, etc.

BAY LAUREL *Laurus nobilis*

Associated with the sun, the element fire, and with courage and nobility, bay laurel was known as 'Daphne' to the Greeks, after the nymph who escaped the amorous intentions of Apollo by being transformed into a bay tree. It is held sacred to Apollo, the god of music and poetry, and from this derives the British title 'Poet Laureate' and the term 'to gain one's laurels'. A wreath or crown of bay leaves was used to crown Greek poets, heroes and victors, notably at the Olympic games.

Asclepius, the god of medicine, was also depicted crowned with laurel. The incense of bay was also reputed to have been used by the Delphic priestesses, and was thus associated with the gifts of prophecy, healing and clairvoyance. It was thought that placing the leaves beneath a pillow encouraged divination through dreams.

To the Romans, bay was a symbol of resurrection, because its leaves do not fall or wither, and they hung a wreath on their doorways at New Year to bring good luck. During a time of plague, Emperor Claudius and his court moved to Laurentium, famous for its bay trees, due to their reputation for resisting the spread of contagious epidemics. The Romans also used the scent of bay as a household air freshener or disinfectant and its sweet smell was used to induce sleep.

In the Middle Ages it was thought to be a protection from evil and it is still traditional to plant a bay tree by the door of a house: 'Neither witch nor devil, thunder nor lightening, will hurt a man where a bay tree is.'[7]

A packet of bay laurel given to a bride ensured a long and happy union. It was also used as a stewing herb in Elizabethan times, and its leaves were used in the kitchen to keep weevils and insects away.

It was formerly used for a variety of complaints in herbal medicine, including the treatment of hysteria and nervous afflictions, being 'sovereign against cold diseases of the brain, nerves, joynts and loins'.[8]

SCENT:
Fresh, medicinal, penetrating, slightly camphoraceous, spicy. It blends well with clary sage, cypress, frankincense, juniper, lavender, pine, rosemary, spice and citrus oils.

KEY QUALITIES:
Antiseptic, clearing, inspirational, protective, strengthening, tonic, warming.

CONTRA-INDICATIONS:
Avoid during pregnancy. Narcotic in large doses, may cause headaches: use in moderation only. May cause sensitization in some individuals when applied to the skin.

The essential oil helps clear congestion, fights infection and strengthens the nerves. It is stimulating in small doses and sedative in larger doses, having a warm yet fresh quality.

This oil is suited to writers, poets, painters, musicians and creative artists of all types – those with psychic tendencies who depend on intuition and inspiration for their work. It promotes confidence, insight and courage – which are needed to complete any innovatory project.

N.B. To be distinguished from the West Indian bay (*Myrcia acris*), which is known locally as *bois d'Inde*.

Applications & Methods of Use:

- Use up to 5 drops in the bath for insomnia, nervousness, respiratory congestion and other stress-related disorders.
- The incense is good for creative work and visualization exercises – add a few drops to a vaporizer.
- The vaporized oil makes a pleasing room fragrance and may be used to prevent the spread of infection.

BENZOIN *Styrax benzoin*

The name of this aromatic resin derives from the Arabic *luban-jawi*, meaning 'incense from Sumatra', and indeed it has been used as a medicine and fragrance by many cultures for thousands of years.

In 1476, the Sultan of Egypt, Melech Elmazda, sent the Queen of Cyprus a present of 15 *rotoli* (about 40 kg) of benzoin, showing its value in the ancient world. It was held in high regard by the Greeks and Romans, who called it respectively *Silphion* and *Laserpitium*. They included the powdered resin in pot pourris, due to its fine fragrance and good fixative properties.

The Portuguese navigator Barboza was thought to have introduced benzoin to Europe in the sixteenth century and it was first known in English as 'benjoin'. In 1623 the British set up a factory in Siam to produce it, such was its popularity.

Ruled by the sun, the gum was considered 'heating and drying … a good cephalic comforting the brain by its grateful smell'.[9] Elizabeth I carried a pomander of ambergris and benzoin.

In France it was called *baume pulmon-aire*, pulmonary balsam, because the fumes helped combat respiratory infections and asthma, and prevent the spread of contagious disease.

In the East, the fumigations were believed to drive away evil spirits. It is still employed as an incense for Buddhist and Hindu worship, and in India it is burned by the wealthy classes for pleasure. At religious ceremonies, Muslim women burn incense made of benzoin, aloe wood, sandalwood and patchouli. When burned at the feet of the dead, the fragrance is believed to lift the soul to heaven.

The essential oil warms and stimulates the heart and circulation both physically and metaphorically, yet has a soothing, elevating effect on the mind. Eventually it has a soporific effect.

> This essence creates a kind of euphoria; it interposes a padded zone between us and events.[10]

Benzoin is good for people who are cut off from their heart and their feelings, either due to their temperament or to an emotional hurt or shock, for it helps to melt away blockages. Known as 'benjamin' in the perfume trade, it is also the main ingredient in one of the world's most popular perfumes, 'Chypres'.

SCENT:
Balsamic, intense, resinous, rich, sweet, vanilla-like. It blends well with coriander, cypress, frankincense, jasmine, juniper, lemon, myrrh, rose, sandalwood and other spicy oils.

KEY QUALITIES:
Comforting, elevating, energizing, fixative, preservative, purifying, stimulating (heart and circulation), uplifting, warming.

CONTRA-INDICATIONS:
May cause allergic reaction when applied to the skin in some individuals.

N.B. Storax (*Liquidambar orientalis*) has similar properties to benzoin. It is also an ancient aromatic material, highly valued in the East as an incense and perfume fixative.

APPLICATIONS & METHODS OF USE:

- Use 5–10 drops in the bath for emotional and physical exhaustion, nervous anxiety, grief, depression, loneliness and feelings of loss.
- The vaporized oil makes a warm and comforting room fragrance. The inhaled fumes are beneficial for all catarrh and chest infections, sinusitis, asthma etc.; also to ward off colds, 'flu or other infections.
- Benzoin makes a good addition to a massage oil for emotional complaints – e.g. 2 drops each of rose, orange and benzoin in 1 Tbs sweet almond oil rubbed clockwise into the solar plexus and chest area.

- Use the oil in pot pourris, to perfume linen and in herb pillows.
- The incense is conducive to meditation or prayer; it helps to evoke a peaceful, alert state of mind.

BERGAMOT *Citrus bergamia*

SCENT:
Citrus, fresh, green, light, slightly spicy floral, sweet, warm.
It blends well with most oils, notably cedar, clary sage, cypress, geranium, jasmine, lavender, melissa, neroli and other citrus oils.

KEY QUALITIES:
Anti-depressant, antiseptic, balancing, calming, encouraging, healing, insect repellent, protective, refreshing, regulating, reviving, sedative (nervous system), soothing, uplifting.

CONTRA-INDICATIONS:
Phototoxic – unless it is a bergapten-free oil (which should be stated on the bottle) do not apply to skin which may be exposed to the sun's rays as it causes discoloration.

The bergamot tree is said to have been introduced to the New World from the Canary Islands by Christopher Columbus. By the sixteenth century the essence was already widely known throughout Europe and is mentioned in many old manuscripts and herbals.

In the West it reached a height of popularity during the time of Napoleon, usually mixed with otto of neroli and rosemary in the form of eau de cologne, or simply as a reviving essence mixed with rectified spirits and applied to handkerchiefs. In Voodoo, the essence is used to protect from misfortune and physical danger; it is also used to anoint the heads of all participants during initiation rituals!

Bergamot has long been used as a traditional Italian folk remedy, especially for fever and infection. Recent studies have shown that the oil effectively balances the activity of the hypothalamus. The essential oil has a soothing effect on the nervous system, yet the light, fresh, citrus fragrance has an uplifting effect on the mind. It can therefore stimulate or sedate according to individual needs.

> In helping with mental and psychological states, bergamot is almost the most valuable oil at the aromatherapist's disposal.[11]

It is especially good for those who have a propensity towards depression, who suffer from negative thoughts and find it difficult to motivate themselves or change their pattern of behaviour. Paoli Rovesti, while conducting research in psychiatric units, found that bergamot oil had important psychological effects on patients: it helped relieve fear and calm anxiety. Rovesti also recommended bergamot oil for people who want to give up smoking. To sum up:

> With its many layered effects, bergamot remains uplifting. For exhaustion when convalescing from physical or psychological illness or for fatigue due to constant stress, this essential oil stimulates and helps rebuild strength. It helps calm people under stress or who feel nervous or anxious … the oil helps people regain self-confidence, and it uplifts and refreshes the spirit.[12]

APPLICATIONS & METHODS OF USE:

- Put 5–10 drops in the bath for stress, depression, grief, anxiety, despondency and PMT.
- Bergamot blends well with cypress, geranium, lavender or neroli for use in massage oil blends, e.g. 2 drops each of bergamot, lavender and neroli in 1 Tbs sweet almond oil.
- Used regularly in the bath or oil burners it can help to regulate the appetite and is therefore good for obesity or anorexia.
- The delightful scent of the vaporized oil helps prevent the spread of germs in the atmosphere and creates a pleasing, uplifting fragrance in the home. It combines well with myrtle.
- The scent may also be used to keep insects at bay. Keep cats and dogs away from plants by using a few drops in a plant spray every few days.

CAMPHOR *Cinnamomum camphora*

Camphor was known to medieval alche-mists as a watery cold substance under the domination of the moon. There has been disagreement about whether it is warming or cooling, since it seems to have an initial cooling effect followed by a rubefacient or burning sensation, and it tends to react to individual needs.

Camphor was once commonly worn in a small pouch around the neck to ward off colds, 'flu and other infections, and its fragrance was used by the Arabs to lessen sexual desire. It was also used to calm hysteria, nervous excitement and neuralgia – and, on the other hand, used for heart failure.

> This balancing effect is also apparent in its effect on the nervous system. It stimulates languid depression and sedates hysteria; it is of use in most psychosomatic or nervous diseases. Camphor will often produce results where milder remedies are insufficiently effective, or when a gentle shock is required in order to produce some reaction from a chronically sick body.[13]

Camphor stimulates the heart, circulation and lungs, yet sedates the nervous system. According to Grieve, it stimulates the brain and the intellect. The smell repels insects, moths and worms, so it was the original component of moth balls.

Borneo camphor (*Dryobalanops aromatica*), which is less toxic, has an odour which is reminiscent of

SCENT:
Camphoraceous, clear, penetrating, pungent, sharp. Blends well with spicy and herbal oils.

KEY QUALITIES:
Analgesic (pain-killing), anaphrodisiac, balancing (extremes of heat or cold), restorative.

CONTRA-INDICATIONS:
In its crude form camphor is extremely poisonous – only the 'white' camphor, the lightest fraction, should be used; brown or yellow camphor should not be used in therapy. White camphor is relatively safe, but use in moderation only, due to toxicity levels. Homeopathic remedies are negated by the vapours alone. It should be avoided by epileptics.

patchouli and labdanum, and has similar properties to camphor. It has been used since the earliest times in the East as a medicine, for embalming purposes and as an incense. Borneo camphor is still popular, especially in China, where it is used to scent soap and as an incense at funerals.

APPLICATIONS & METHODS OF USE:

- The vaporized oil can be used for shock, nervousness, worrying thoughts, depression, apathy, or over-excitement. It is also a good insect repellent.

CARAWAY *Carum carvi*

Remains of fossilized caraway seeds have been found in Neolithic dwelling-sites, which show that it was being used some 8,000 years ago. Ancient Egyptian papyrus documents dated 25000 BC record that caraway was used as an incense in early religious ceremonies and in perfumes.

It was well known throughout the early Arab world and it is probable that the English name derives from the old Arabic term *Karawya*, which is still in use in the East today.

The classical Roman and Greek writers mention the use of caraway frequently – Dioscorides advised the oil to be taken by 'pale-faced girls'. The Romans ate the seeds after meals to sweeten the breath and, like the Arabs and later the Central Europeans and Scandinavians especially, they used them as an aromatic ingredient in cakes and bread. Julius Caesar refers to *chara*, a type of bread made from caraway roots mixed with milk that was

SCENT:
Anise-like, strong, sweet spicy, warm.
It blends well with cinnamon, jasmine, lavender, rose and other spices.

KEY QUALITIES:
Antiseptic, cleansing, insect repellent, protective, restorative, stimulating, strengthening, tonic (for the nervous system), warming.

CONTRA-INDICATIONS:
May cause dermal irritation in concentration – use in low dilution only.

eaten by the soldiers of Valerius. The Germans and Russians make a liqueur from the seeds, known as *Kummel*.

According to Culpeper, caraway is a spice under Mercury whose 'seed is conducing to all cold griefs of the head and stomach'. Indeed, it was thought to strengthen the mind and spirit, and recommended for symptoms attending hysteria and other nervous disorders, especially nervous dyspepsia.

Caraway was also thought to confer the gift of retention, i.e. 'preventing the theft of any object which contained it, and holding the thief in custody within the invaded house'.[14] In the same way, it was believed to keep lovers from proving fickle (thus forming a common ingredient of love potions), and also to prevent fowls and pigeons from straying.

A few seeds placed under a child's mattress were also thought to protect from illness, nightmares or evil spirits. The seeds, tied in muslin bags, have also been used historically to scent drawers and clothes, and to keep moths away. Napoleon is said to have favoured caraway-scented soap.

In medical herbalism caraway is valued as a digestive remedy, especially for nervous dyspepsia. In aromatherapy, it is used for its tonic effect on the nervous system and for its clean, stimulating scent.

APPLICATIONS & METHODS OF USE:

- Add up to 5 drops to the bath to help combat mental fatigue, strain, exhaustion, nervous dyspepsia and general weakness.
- As a massage oil, it is best used in combination with other tonic essences, e.g. 2 drops each of caraway, rosemary and lavender in 1 Tbs base oil.
- As a vaporized oil it makes a pleasing, uplifting room fragrance or incense. It also keeps insects at bay.
- The oil may be added to pot pourris, used to scent linen or clothes and, in minute amounts, employed in home perfumes.

CARDAMOM 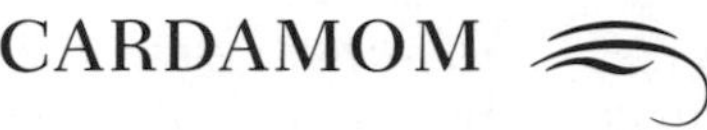 *Elettoria cardamomum*

Known and used since the earliest times, cardamom is mentioned by Dioscorides, Pliny, Theophrastus and Pomet. Plutarch recorded in the first century AD that it was used by the ancient Egyptians in their religious ceremonies and in perfumes. It was also included in their 'Metopion' ointment, which was considered generally mollifying, and heat and sweat producing. According to Dioscorides, the best 'Metopion' was the one that smelt more of cardamom and myrrh than of galbanum. It was also included in the Egyptian recipe for 'Oil of Lilies'. In Greek and Roman times it was favoured for use mainly in perfumery: Ovid and other poets praised cardamom's pleasing aroma.

The plant has been used in Eastern traditional medicine for over 3,000 years, being mentioned in the Vedic medical texts under the name 'Ela'. Its main reputation in India, however, is as a powerful aphrodisiac. The powdered seeds are also used in the preparation of incense and fumigating powders, together with cascarilla and sandalwood. Cardamom, cloves, curcuma and sandalwood are blended to form a special powder known as 'Abir', which is used as an incense during Hindu ceremonies.

Cardamom is included in the Tibetan preparation 'Aquilaria A', whose medicated fumes are inhaled for stress-related conditions including insomnia, anxiety, nervous tension and hysteria amongst others.

The Arabs sometimes add a few seeds to their coffee for their pleasing aroma and cardamom features several times in *The Arabian Nights*. An Arabian aphrodisiac recommended by Shaykh Nafzawi included cardamom, cinnamon, cloves, nutmeg, pepper and gillyflowers, and was to be taken night and morning.

Known in Europe as 'Fire of Venus', car-

> SCENT:
> *Pleasing, powerful, soft, spicy, sweet, warm. High odour intensity – easily overshadows other smells.*
> *Blends well with floral fragrances in minute amounts.*
>
> KEY QUALITIES:
> *Antiseptic, aphrodisiac, cephalic, comforting, nerve and heart tonic, penetrating, refreshing, soothing, stimulant, uplifting, warming.*

damom was once used in medieval love potions. In Victorian England, it was common to nibble the seeds as sweetmeats. The scent neutralizes the smell of garlic and in various cultures the seeds have often been chewed after meals to sweeten the breath.

Mrs Grieve recommended cardamom for 'disorders of the head' and Mme Maury considered it good for those with a weak heart due to emotional problems.

> It may not have a physiological effect on the nervous system, but it certainly has psychological effect, and is especially good for digestive problems of nervous origin.[15]

It has a warm, soft, pervasive aroma which has a uplifting yet soothing effect on the mind and spirits. It is also a cephalic.

APPLICATIONS & METHODS OF USE:

- An excellent, refreshing yet soothing bath oil, best blended with other oils. Use for headaches, mental fatigue, anxiety, stress, insomnia, debility and nervous weakness of all types.
- For an aphrodisiac, restorative massage oil, add a few drops of cardamom to a sensual blend of essences such as jasmine, sandalwood and neroli.
- Use as an uplifting incense or as a room freshener, especially to help eliminate the smell of cigarette smoke or other unwanted odours.
- Cardamom makes a long-lasting addition to pot pourris, herb pillows and to an individual perfume – but take care to use only a little since the scent tends to overwhelm other fragrances.

CEDARWOOD ATLAS  *Cedrus atlantica*

This is closely related to the famous cedar of Lebanon which the ancient Egyptians considered to be imperishable. They used it to entomb human bodies, to make the doors to their temples and to build ships. The fragrant wood was burned in the temples and the oil was injected into corpses during the mummification process. It was also used in remedies and perfumes, including the famous 'mithridat', an antidote to poisons.

Solomon's Temple was constructed exclusively of Lebanese cedarwood, as was his chariot, as documented in the 'Song of Solomon'. Cedar is frequently mentioned in the Bible, and was used to symbolize everything that was fertile, abundant and noble or had great spiritual strength, from the Arabic *kedron* or *kedree*, meaning 'power'.

Also closely related to the Atlas cedarwood is yellow cedar, known as 'The Tree of Life'. Its oil, which is called 'thuja', is derived from the Greek word meaning 'to fumigate' or *thuo*, to sacrifice, for the fragrant wood was burned by the ancients at sacrifices.

Horace speaks of books preserved with cedarwood oil and of keeping documents in cedar chests – hence the ancient proverb 'worthy of being cased in cedar'. Dioscorides and Galen mention that the resin from the cedar preserved the body from putrefaction, and so it was called 'the life of him that is dead'.

Herodotus records the use of cedarwood oil by Assyrian women, mixed with cypress and frankincense and used as an anointing oil. Resin from the Indian or deodar cedar is still used as a temple incense in Tibet and by Tibetan exiles in India.

SCENT:
Balsamic, dry woody, pleasing, slightly camphoraceous, smoky, sweet, tenacious, turpentine-like. It blends well with bergamot, cassia, clary sage, cypress, frankincense, jasmine, juniper, mimosa, neroli, rosemary, vetiver and ylang ylang.

KEY QUALITIES:
Antiseptic, aphrodisiac, comforting, elevating, fixative, grounding, long-lasting, opening, preservative, protective, rejuvenating, stimulant, strengthening, tonic, vermifuge, warming.

CONTRA-INDICATIONS:
Best avoided during pregnancy.

The essential oil of the Atlas cedar has a tenacious aroma which has a stimulating, elevating and opening effect on the mind and psyche. It has a strong, life-giving quality, which helps relieve anxiety and quell anger, irritation or fear.

N.B. The oil from the so-called Virginian cedarwood (*Juniperus virginiana*), which has a soft, pencil-wood fragrance, and Texas cedarwood (*J. mexicana*), which has a 'tar-like odour', should not be used as substitutes for Atlas cedarwood oil therapeutically.

APPLICATIONS & METHODS OF USE:

- Use 5–10 drops in the bath for exhaustion, nervous tension, anger and other stress-related complaints, for it is reviving to the body and uplifting and comforting to the mind.
- Blends well with other woody oils for massage, especially for stress.
- Vaporize the oil as an incense for meditation, yoga or prayer: it helps clear the head and deepen the breath. Good as a warming, refreshing room fragrance, for creating a sensual mood or as an insect repellent. Research has also shown that cedarwood and pine are very effective in eliminating unwanted odours.
- May be used neat as a woody 'masculine' scent and added to pot pourris or linen to protect against moths, etc.

CHAMOMILE  *Matricaria chamomilla* and *Anthemis nobilis*

There are several species of chamomile which share similar properties and characteristics, but the most commonly used are the Roman or sweet chamomile (*Anthemis*), and the German type (*Matricaria*), also commonly known as 'Chamomile Blue' due to its characteristic inky blue colour.

Roman chamomile has been used for over 2,000 years, especially throughout the Mediterranean region. Its name derives from the Greek *kamai melon*, meaning ground apple, because its strong fruity scent resembles that of fallen apples. It was held sacred by the ancient Egyptians who dedicated it to the sun god Ra; the aromatic oil was also used in Egypt as a medicine for all types of ague (intermittent fever), and was used for anointing the body from head to foot. It was also valued highly by the Arab physicians and appears in many Moorish herbals. It was called 'Maythen' by the Saxons and revered as one of their nine sacred herbs. It was later dedicated to St Anne, mother of the Virgin Mary.

Edward III used chamomile to scent his clothes and linen, while the Elizabethans used camomile as a strewing herb and as a fumigant to rid homes of 'the foulness of offending odours'. During the Tudor period the chamomile lawn became popular, grown for its sturdy growth and delicious, aromatic fragrance when it was stepped on.

In the language of flowers, chamomile stands for 'patience in adversity', due to its delicate but hardy nature. It was once used a great deal in the treatment of hysteria, melancholy and nervous afflictions of all types, especially women's ailments. It is still recommended in the *British Herbal Pharmacopoeia* for nervous dyspepsia, restlessness and irritability in children.

SCENT:
Fresh, grassy, herbaceous, rich, slightly fruity, sweet, warm. The German chamomile has an intense, slightly bitter odour compared to the more fragrant, apple-like scent of the Roman type. They blend well with patchouli, lavender, clary sage, jasmine, geranium, neroli, rose, benzoin and citrus oils.

KEY QUALITIES:
Analgesic, antiseptic, balancing, comforting, healing, mild, relaxing, restorative, sedative, slightly soporific or hypnotic in large doses, soothing, tonic, warming.

It is a useful mild sedative for children, having a calming but not a depressing effect. It is also a good oil for helping to deal with underlying emotional difficulties that often manifest as skin problems such as eczema, rashes or allergies.

Chamomile has a profoundly calming effect on the emotional level, so it is very helpful for people who tend be hyperactive, workaholic, think too much and worry a lot. Also for hyper-sensitive individuals who are deeply affected by emotional upsets, especially those prone to allergies. Both oils, but especially the German type, stimulate the immune system.

N.B. Chamomile Maroc (*Ormenis mixta*), with a rosy-honey fragrance, belongs to a related but distinct family and, although a useful oil in perfumery, does not have the same associations or therapeutic value as the 'true' camomiles.

APPLICATIONS & METHODS OF USE:

- Use up to 10 drops in the bath for nervous afflictions of all types, including headaches, insomnia, migraine, PMT, dizziness, restlessness, anxiety, menopausal problems, nervous depression and irritability. Excellent for children's sleeplessness, tantrums, weepiness or over-excitement (5 drops only).
- As a massage oil (6 drops in 1 Tbs sweet almond oil), chamomile also acts as a restorative to the nervous system; good for nervous exhaustion, weariness and overcoming stress. Blends well with bergamot, clary sage, geranium, jasmine, lavender, neroli and rose.
- During pregnancy, to help overcome restlessness, fear or anxiety, blend chamomile, rose and lavender together for use in massage, burners or the bath.
- A few drops can be put on the pillow, on night clothes or used in the bedroom at night in a burner (in a safe place) for insomnia or restlessness.
- Inhaling the fumes by putting a few drops on a hanky or in a burner helps combat emotional anxiety and tension associated with asthma, hayfever and other allergies. The vaporized oil also acts as a disinfectant to help stop the spread of infections such as colds, flu, etc.
- Chamomile tea is a traditional soothing night-cap, useful for both adults and children. Use a dessertspoonful of dried flowers to a pint (600 ml) boiling water, let steep and sweeten with honey.
- The oil can be added to perfumes, pot pourris and herb pillows, and used as a clothes freshener, for it gives a pleasing, soothing aroma.

CINNAMON — *Cinnamomum zeylanicum*

Cinnamon has been used continually since ancient times, and was one of the oldest and most valuable items in the spice trade. The Egyptians used cinnamon as a medicine and as incense and perfume material. It was included in the recipe for the famous remedy 'Megaleion' and in the perfume *par excellence* known as 'The Egyptian' as well as in 'Kyphi'. It was one of the principal spices used in the mummification process and was considered valuable enough to be presented to the temple as a gift.

It is mentioned in the Bible on several occasions and was included in the holy ointment of Moses:

> Take thou unto thee principal spices, of pure myrrh five hundred shekels, and of sweet cinnamon half so much – and thou shalt make it an oil of holy ointment.[16]

The Arabs valued cinnamon, for to them it was a symbol of wealth; they used the oil to anoint the sacred vessels used in their religious ceremonies. For centuries the Arabs kept the source of cinnamon a closely guarded secret, but it is said that Alexander the Great perceived that he was near the coast of Arabia when his ship was enveloped by the scent of fragrant spices wafting from the shore.

Pliny used cinnamon in a perfume recipe for men in his *Natural History*, and many sources recommend it as a spice with which to perfume linen, since it keeps moths away.

In Chinese medicine, cinnamon was seen as something of a cure-all and few recipes were complete without it. It was employed as a nerve tranquillizer and

> SCENT:
> *Dry, hot, peppery, slightly woody, sweet spicy, tenacious. It blends well with benzoin, frankincense, myrrh, orange and ylang ylang.*
>
> KEY QUALITIES:
> *Analgesic, antiseptic, aphrodisiac, protective, restorative, stimulant, strengthening, tonic, uplifting, warming.*
>
> CONTRA-INDICATIONS:
> *Use only cinnamon leaf oil in moderation – cinnamon bark oil is a severe skin irritant.*

tonic, and considered good for depression and a weak heart. In the East generally, the powdered bark was a common ingredient of incense and fumigating preparations.

Cinnamon was brought to Western Europe at the time of the Crusades, where it was used in medicines and perfumes as well as for flavouring food. It was given to the melancholic, the sick and elderly especially. All over medieval Europe it was considered an aphrodisiac and included in love potions:

> Upon inhalation, the oil is reported to act as a sexual stimulant to the female.[17]

Dr Valnet prescribes an aphrodisiac wine containing 30 g vanilla, 30 g cinnamon, 30 g ginseng and 30 g rhubarb in 1 litre of Malaga wine or mature Chablis![18]

N.B. Cassia (*Cinnamomum cassia*) or Chinese cinnamon is closely related and also has a long history of use for similar purposes.

APPLICATIONS & METHODS OF USE:

- Use up to 5 drops in the bath for nausea, faintness, debility, depression, nervous exhaustion and other stress-related conditions.
- For massage, it is best used in combination with other essences, such as 2 drops each of cinnamon, frankincense and orange in 1 Tbs sweet almond oil.
- As an aphrodisiac, it is good as an ingredient in a sensual massage oil blend, perfume or room fragrance.
- As a vaporized oil it helps clear the head, disperse unwanted smells and prevent the spread of infection. Effective as an uplifting incense for meditation, yoga, etc.
- May also be used in pot pourris and to scent linen and clothes.

CLARY SAGE

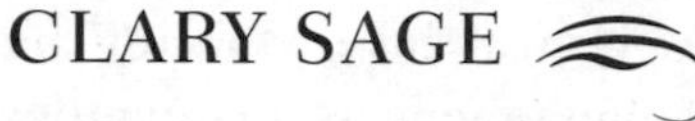

see Sage

CLOVE *Eugenia caryophyllata*

For a long time, cloves were the most expensive of all the spices and held in high regard. They were thought of as a general panacea and were most probably used as such by the ancient Egyptians.

Cloves were also known in China as early as 266 BC, when it was customary for subjects of the court to hold the spice in their mouth while addressing the sovereign so their breath had a pleasant odour. In Chinese medicine, cloves are considered a warming agent, good for hypertension. They are still used in the Tibetan remedy 'Aquilaria A' as a stress-relieving agent for anxiety, tension, hysteria, insomnia, etc.

It is thought that the Arabs were the first to trade in cloves after they discovered the Molucca islands off the north coast of Africa, where the first wild clove trees grew. On Molucca, it is still traditional for girls to wear clove flowers, and children are given necklaces of clove seeds as amulets to preserve them from illness and the 'evil eye'. Later, cloves were brought to the Mediterranean ports by the Persians, Arabians and Egyptians. The strongly aromatic seeds were also regarded as aphrodisiac.

Pliny praised cloves, as did the Roman doctor Alexander Trallianus. St Hildegarde, in her book *Morborum Causae et Curae*, recommended cloves for the treatment of headaches and migraines.

In Europe during the Middle Ages, pom-anders were made with cloves to

SCENT:
Fragrant, fresh, fruity, hot, peppery, sweet spicy.
Blends well with bergamot, caraway, geranium, lavender, orange, rose and ylang ylang.

KEY QUALITIES:
Analgesic, antiseptic, aphrodisiac, comforting, purifying, revitalizing, soothing, stimulating, tonic, warming.

CONTRA-INDICATIONS:
Use only clove bud in moderation. Clove leaf and clove stem cause skin irritation.

keep epidemics, especially the plague, at bay. This was the basis for the practice, still in use today, of sticking cloves in an orange as a pomander to sweeten the wardrobe and linen and keep moths away.

Oil of cloves is best known today in the West as a toothache remedy. However, it has other household uses, as Danielle Ryman writes:

> When I am under physical or mental strain, or simply tired, I suck a clove several times a day. It has an agreeable taste, and acts as a relaxant. Sucking cloves is a particularly good idea for those trying to give up smoking.[19]

APPLICATION & METHODS OF USE:

- Use up to 3 drops, together with other essences, in the bath or in a body oil for physical and intellectual weakness, convalescence, frigidity, poor memory and stress-related complaints.
- Good for creating a warm, sensual and festive mood.
- The vaporized oil helps clear the head, purify the air and prevent the spread of germs.
- Use the oil or cloves in pot pourris, linen bags or in individual perfumes.

CORIANDER *Coriandrum sativum*

The fruits have been used as a spice since the earliest times, as a medicine and in perfumes. Coriander was employed mainly as a remedy by the ancient Egyptians and according to Pliny was used as an antidote to the 'two headed serpent, the amphisbaena'. An unguent containing coriander, dill, bryony and donkey's fat was used to treat headaches while the mixture of fresh garlic and coriander in wine was considered a potent aphrodisiac, which also had the power to bring happiness! Another reference cites coriander as promoting a good night's sleep. It was among the herbs offered to the temple by the king, and its seeds were found in the tomb of Tutankhamun and Rameses II. An oil from the seeds was used in religious ceremonies.

Coriander is common in the Holy Land, and is mentioned in the

Bible on several occasions, being likened to the manna that the Lord provided for the children of Israel. It was one of the bitter herbs designated to be eaten at Passover. In India it has been used for thousands of years in curries and also for religious ritual. It has been employed by the Chinese for over 5,000 years and was believed to promote longevity. It is still used as a tonic for the stomach and heart, and to deaden pain. It also has a long history of use by the Arabs and appears as an aphrodisiac in *The Arabian Nights*. It is still taken by Arab women to ease the pain of labour.

The Greeks and Romans were familiar with coriander, which they used mainly as a flavouring. Dioscorides claimed it was a 'calmant' and Galen praised it as a tonic. Throughout Europe it was formerly held to be an aphrodisiac and an aid to the memory. It was thought of as a witch's plant and in medieval times it was an ingredient of love potions. In the Middle Ages it was put in the popular drink 'Hippocras', which was a feature of Tudor weddings and other festivities, to help raise the spirits.

SCENT:
Anisey, fresh, slightly musky, sweet spicy, woody. The fresh seeds lose their disagreeable scent on drying.
Coriander blends well with bergamot, clary, cypress, frankincense, jasmine, neroli, petitgrain, pine, sandalwood and other spicy oils.

KEY QUALITIES:
Analgesic, aphrodisiac, comforting, purifying, refreshing, revitalizing, soothing, soporific (in excess), stimulating, strengthening, warming.

CONTRA-INDICATIONS:
Use in moderation only, narcotic in excess.

According to Meunier:

> The juice of freshly picked plants when ingested in weak doses has properties similar to those of alcohol: it excites and then depresses. Larger doses lead to manic drunkenness, and eventual prostration.[20]

A similar pattern appears to be the result of inhaling the fumes in excess. The scent of coriander has an initial stimulating effect on the nervous system, but can eventually lead to a soporific effect with over-exposure. Danielle Ryman recommends it for 'headaches and sometimes depression, providing it is used in small quantities'.[21]

The famous toilet water first produced by the Carmelites in Paris during the seventeenth century owes much of its success to coriander. In Victorian and Edwardian times the seeds were chewed after meals to aid digestion and sweeten the breath.

APPLICATIONS & METHODS OF USE:

- For a good refreshing bath oil, add up to 5 drops to the bath. Useful for fatigue, depression, nervous exhaustion, PMT, migraine, headaches and other stress-related complaints.
- Use as a vaporized oil to purify the air of germs and as an uplifting yet calming room fragrance. Helps create a sensual mood.
- Use in combination with other essences in a massage oil for a reviving, soothing and aphrodisiac blend.
- The seeds may be used in pot pourris, the oil added to individual perfumes.

CYPRESS  *Cupressus sempervirens*

Cypress was highly valued as an incense and medicine by early civilizations. The ancient Egyptians used the wood to make their sarcophagi and it was also used as an incense by the Assyrians. A variety of cypress is still burned by the Tibetans as a purification incense. The word *sempervirens* means 'ever-living', and the ancient Greeks, Romans and Egyptians dedicated the tree to their gods of the Underworld. It is frequently grown in cemeteries, and one of its folk names is 'The Tree of Death', though it symbolically represents life after death. In Western magic, ritual objects are consecrated in its smoke, and the oil is used for blessing and protection.

> The smoke of the leaves drives away gnats, the shavings of the wood preserves from moth and the rosin is laid among garments.[22]

In medical herbalism, it is best known as a styptic and astringent. In *Subtle Aromatherapy*, Patricia Davis writes:

> Cypress oil is helpful at times of transition, such as career changes, moving home or major spiritual decisions such as changing one's religion … bereavement or the ending of a close relationship.[23]

According to Valnet it is a good general tonic, especially of the nervous system. It sedates the nerve endings, but is uplifting to the spirit.

The essential oil also helps balance the female hormonal system, making it valuable for PMT or menopausal problems.

SCENT:
Austere, balsamic, dry, slightly nutty, smoky, spicy, sweet, tenacious, woody. Blends well with benzoin, bergamot, chamomile, clary sage, lavender, lemon, orange, rose, wood and spicy oils.

KEY QUALITIES:
Antiseptic, astringent, comforting, drying, protective, purifying, refreshing, regulating, relaxing, restorative, reviving, soothing, warming.

APPLICATIONS & METHODS OF USE:

- Add 5–10 drops to the bath for PMT, menopausal problems, irritability, nervous tension, anxiety and stress-related problems.
- Best blended with other oils for massage, e.g. 2 drops each of cypress, Atlas cedarwood and rose in 1 Tbs sweet almond oil.
- The vaporized oil clears the head, kills germs and is good as a purifying incense. Keeps insects at bay.
- May be used neat as a perfume and in pot pourris, etc.

ELEMI *Canarium luzonicum*

One of the aromatics used by the ancient Egyptians for embalming, cosmetics and perfumes. It was also used throughout the Arab and Turkish world in ancient times. Its name in Arabic means 'above and below', a shortened version of the old kabalistic and alchemical term 'as above, so below', referring to the correspondence between the spiritual and earthly realms.

Introduced into Europe in the fifteenth century, elemi was used as an

> SCENT:
> *Balsamic, fresh, incense-like, light, slightly camphoraceous, soft, spicy.*
> *It blends well with clary sage, frankincense, lavender, myrrh, rosemary and spicy oils.*
>
> KEY QUALITIES:
> *Drying, fortifying, healing, preserving, restorative, stimulating, warming.*

ingredient in numerous balms, unguents and liniments, due to its ability to speed up the healing process. Heating and drying, it was also used for all types of cold and contracted conditions:

> The distilled oile, as the resin, is specific in all affections of the nerves, palsies and spasms.[24]

Of elemi's psychological effects, Patricia Davis writes:

> The oil has a unifying effect ... Elemi brings feelings of deep peacefulness combined with complete lucidity ... It is helpful for all types of meditation, but seems particularly to enhance visualization.[25]

APPLICATIONS & METHODS OF USE:

- Add 5–10 drops to the bath for stress-related conditions, such as nervous tension, irritability, anxiety and depression.
- Use the vaporized oil as an incense for meditation or as refreshing room fragrance.
- Add to personal perfumes, pot pourris, massage lotions, etc., for its preserving, fixative properties.

EUCALYPTUS BLUE GUM *Eucalyptus globulus*

Eucalyptus was a traditional remedy of the Australian and Tasmanian natives, especially for healing wounds, reducing fever and combating infection. The aborigines used the burning leaves in the form of a fumigation, by seating the sick by the smoke from the fire. In Australia, it is still widely used as a household remedy 'where at the first sign of any sickness, decoctions would be kept simmering as a fumigant on the stove, twenty-four hours a day'.[26] The dried leaves were also smoked like cigarettes for asthma and bronchitis.

A specimen of the blue gum was first brought back to Europe from Tasmania by the famous French naturalist Labillardière in 1793. Labillardière made invaluable observations on the natives and their simple life-style, including the folk use of eucalyptus.

SCENT:
Fresh, penetrating, slightly sweet, woody camphoraceous. It blends well with lavender, lemon, pine, rosemary and thyme.

KEY QUALITIES:
Analgesic, antiseptic, balancing, balsamic, clearing, insect repellent, purifying, refreshing, regulating, stimulating.

CONTRA-INDICATIONS:
Apply in dilution only: in concentration, eucalyptus can irritate the skin. In large doses it is a nervous depressant. Should not be used by young children.

In the West it has become well known as a 'vapour rub' for colds, coughs, sinusitis and respiratory ailments in general, also for aches and pains. In India, the oil is used for the treatment of fever and contagious disease. It has a cooling effect on the body, which quickly brings about a drop in temperature. Its powerful odour also has a revitalizing, stimulating effect on the nervous system as a whole. The fresh aroma is good for nervous exhaustion or general sluggishness.

N.B. There are over 500 different types of eucalyptus, some of which, like the citron-scented gum (*E. citriodora*), are used for perfumery, while others, like the broad-leaved peppermint eucalyptus (*E. dives*), are used in industry. The blue gum is used mainly in pharmaceutical preparations, but also in soaps and medicated toiletries. Cajeput, niaouli and tea tree oil share somewhat similar properties.

APPLICATIONS & METHODS OF USE:

- Use up to 3 drops in the bath or in a 1 tsp massage oil base for debility, nervous exhaustion, convalescence, migraine and congested headaches.

- The vaporized oil is excellent for clearing the head, and reviving the mind and spirit. It also repels insects, purifies the air of germs and prevents the spread of infection.
- Apply a few drops to a tissue for use throughout the day to ease congestion or headaches.

FENNEL, SWEET  *Foeniculum dulce*

Sweet fennel is a herb with a long history of use as a medicine and culinary aid, in both Western and Eastern cultures. It is mentioned in Anglo-Saxon herbals and was used by the ancient Egyptians for various ailments. The early Greek athletes ate the seeds to increase their strength while training for the Olympic games. Fennel was also cultivated by the Romans, and gladiators added it to their food to give them stamina and courage. Later it became associated with longevity and good luck.

Mentioned by Pliny, Hippocrates and Dioscorides, it was considered an effective remedy against snake-bite and other poisons. It was also regarded as anti-venomous by the Chinese and Hindus. This anti-toxic property may be why medieval herbalists described fennel as a charm against evil spirits and witchcraft. A sprig of fennel was traditionally hung over the door on Mid-summer's eve to protect the household against the devil. The seed was also placed in keyholes to bar the entrance of ghosts!

SCENT:
Anise-like, earthy, peppery, sweet: its name derives from the Latin foenum, meaning 'hay', due to its musty fragrance.
It blends well with geranium, lavender, rose and sandalwood.

KEY QUALITIES:
Balancing, cleansing, insect repellent, normalizing, purifying, restorative, revitalizing, stimulating.

CONTRA-INDICATIONS:
Should not be used by epileptics, children under six or pregnant women. Narcotic in large doses – use in moderation only.

According to Culpeper, it is a herb of Mercury and under Virgo, being hot, heating and drying. It was believed to be good for the heart and was prescribed for those suffering from stroke.

In the sixteenth century it was used 'to make those lean who are too fat' and in Elizabethan times the seeds were chewed like coriander, as a kind of herbal sweetmeat, to calm the stomach and sweeten the breath.

> The odour has a stimulating effect on the nervous and glandular system. The foliage improves memory and is a tonic for the brain.[27]

Dr Valnet considers it a nervine, although in high doses it can cause convulsions. He also states that the essence makes animals timid.

N.B. Sweet fennel is safer for use therapeutically since it is less toxic and does not cause skin irritation like the bitter type. Bitter fennel (*F. sativum*) is preferred in perfumery work.

APPLICATIONS & METHODS OF USE:

- For an excellent tonic bath, add 5–10 drops to the bath. Good for emotional instability caused by PMT or menopausal problems, also mental weakness, nervous debility and convalescence.
- Add 6 drops of fennel oil to 1 Tbs sweet almond oil for a reviving, purifying massage.
- As a vaporized oil it makes a refreshing room fragrance. It also purifies the air of germs and repels fleas and other insects.
- Use the oil or seeds in pot pourris.

FRANKINCENSE OR OLIBANUM *Boswellia carterii*

A fragrance with strong religious associations and a highly esteemed incense material. Its name derives from the medieval French *franc*, meaning free, pure or abundant, and the Latin *incensum*, to kindle. It is also commonly called olibanum, derived from the Hebrew name *lebonah*, and sometimes referred to as 'real incense'. It was carried from Yemen along the Incense Road in large quantities – in the ancient world the demand for frankincense exceeded myrrh by 5 to 1. It was used extensively by the Egyptians for cosmetics and face masks, but not in the embalming process. Along with other aromatics it was mixed with honey and formed into pellets, which were used to fumigate houses, scent hair and clothing and could also be chewed as a masticatory to sweeten the breath. The resin was burned at religious ceremonies as an incense and used as an ingredient in the famous perfume 'Kyphi'.

There is probably no civilization in the East or West that has not prized frankincense as part of its religious rituals – Egyptian, Persian, Babylonian, Assyrian, Greek, Roman and Hebrew cultures all attached great importance to its use. Its inclusion in Jewish rites was laid down in the thirtieth book of Exodus, for it was included in the recipe for holy incense given to Moses by the Lord. The Jews later decreed that only pure frankincense could be used as holy incense. It was offered to Jesus at his birth, along with myrrh, and is mentioned 22 times in the Bible. Frankincense was burned at the Greek altars at Eleutherae in the Temple of Zeus and Demeter. According to Herodotus, frankincense burned on the altar at the Tower of Babel. It is still employed by the Roman Catholic Church as an offering during the Mass, together with benzoin and storax. It was widely offered as a tribute to divine and political powers: English sovereigns (now the Lord Chamberlain) offer up frankincense on the Feast of the Epiphany on 6 January.

The sweet smoke from the resin was believed to drive out evil spirits from the sick. It was used ritually both for the purification of the body and soul, and as a manifestation of the presence of the divine. Avicenna wrote that 'it strengtheneth the wit and understanding'. Culpeper recommended it for depression and poor memory and to strengthen the nerves.

SCENT:
Balsamic, incense-like, long-lasting, resinous, rich, slightly camporaceous, sweet, woody. It blends well with basil, bergamot, camphor, geranium, lavender, orange, neroli, pine, vetiver and the spicy oils.

KEY QUALITIES:
Cephalic, clearing, fixative, preservative, protective, purifying, restorative, revitalizing, sedative, tonic, uplifting, warming.

Psychologically, frankincense has a soothing and elevating effect, which helps to induce the right frame of mind for meditation or worship, and to create an atmosphere suitably different from that in which mundane occupations are carried out. In 1981 German scientists investigated the effects of inhaling frankincense smoke after altar boys were said to have become emotionally addicted to the substance. They found that when burned it produced *trahydrocannabinole* – a psycho-active substance which expands consciousness.

Frankincense is still widely used in the preparation of incense and fumigating preparations. In aromatherapy, it is valued for its tonic effect on the nervous system, and its calming, relaxing effect on the mind and emotions.

APPLICATIONS & METHODS OF USE:

- Add 5–10 drops to the bath for anxiety, nervous tension, depression and stress-related conditions.
- The vaporized oil is conducive to meditation, yoga or prayer; it helps clear the head and deepen the breath.
- For a relaxing massage, blend 2 drops each of frankincense, orange and neroli in 1 Tbs sweet almond oil.
- Add to home perfume blends, pot pourris, etc. for its rich, long-lasting scent and fixative properties.

GALBANUM *Ferula galbaniflua*

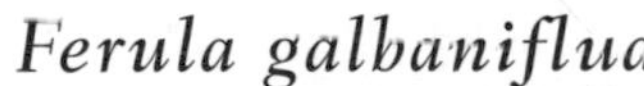

A fragrant greenish gum resin used by ancient civilizations as an incense and medicine, and in Egypt in cosmetics and the embalming process. The 'green incense' mentioned in Egyptian texts may have been galbanum imported from Persia. It was also an ingredient in the famous Mendesian perfume known as 'The Egyptian'.

The Hebrews also used galbanum as an anointing oil and it is referred to in the Bible:

> And the Lord said unto Moses, Take unto thee sweet spices, stacte [nard or storax] and onycha [labdanum], and galbanum; these sweet spices with pure frankincense: of each shall there be a like weight.[28]

SCENT:
Balsamic, green, musky, penetrating, sharp, turpentine-like, woody. It blends well with geranium, lavender, pine, sandalwood, vetiver and ylang ylang.

KEY QUALITIES:
Clearing, healing, insect repellent, purifying, sedative, soothing, uplifting.

Theophrastus mentions that the plant grew in Arcadia, and that the root had warming and healing properties. Dioscorides and Pliny noted its sedative and pain-killing properties. In Coptic medicine it was also was used to expel bugs from the house. Zalou root, a closely related species, is still used in Beirut as an aphrodisiac.

According to Mme Maury, galbanum, along with elemi, signifies 'drying and preservation'.[29] Lovell writes that the essential oil 'heals the hysteric passion, taken or anointed on the navel'.[30]

APPLICATIONS & METHODS OF USE:

- Add 5–10 drops to the bath or in massage oils for nervous tension, anxiety, depression, frigidity and stress-related disorders.
- Use the vaporized oil as an incense for meditation, yoga, etc., to help clear the head; may also be used to repel insects.
- The neat oil may be worn as a perfume, added to pot pourris, etc.

GERANIUM ROSE *Pelargonium graveolens*

There are over 200 species of pelargonium, several of which are used for the extraction of essential oil, such as *P. roseum*, *P. odoratissimum* and *P. capitatum*. The cultivated pelargoniums, which originated in South Africa, should not be confused with the European or American types of wild geranium or cranesbill, although they share similar properties. The botanical name of the genus, 'geranium', is believed to have been used by Dioscorides and is derived from the Greek *geranion* or *geranos*, meaning 'crane', thus 'cranesbill', due to the shape of their seed pods. The pelargonium, likewise, derives its name from the Greek *palargos*, meaning 'stork'.

The species which was used during the medieval period was Herb Robert (*G. robertianum*). It was valued chiefly as a vulnerary and styptic. Like the American cranesbill (*G. maculatum*), it was also regarded as a tonic, good for 'torpor' and 'melancholy'.

In medieval times it was seen as a protective herb, as it says in the old herbal rede:

> Snakes will not go
> where geraniums grow.

According to Culpeper it is a herb of Venus and it was one of the plants which symbolized love. The flowers were once used in herbal love sachets.

SCENT:
Green, floral minty, fresh, rosy sweet, strong.
It blends well with bergamot, clove, jasmine, juniper, lavender, neroli, patchouli, rose, sandalwood and citrus oils.

KEY QUALITIES:
Anti-depressant, balancing, insect repellent, refreshing, stimulates adrenal cortex and lymphatic system, tonic, uplifting.

The pelargonium was first introduced into Europe in 1690 and the cultivation of rose geranium for the production of essential oil was initiated in France in 1847.

In aromatherapy, geranium oil is used for its mild, regulating effect on the nervous system. It makes an excellent tonic and pick-me-up, either as a room fragrance, bath or massage rub, soothing yet revitalizing.

APPLICATIONS & METHODS OF USE:

- Add 5–10 drops to the bath for nervous tension, stress, menopausal problems, PMT, depression, moodiness, debility, convalescence, headache, anxiety, hangover, exhaustion.
- For a restorative, balancing massage oil, blend 2 drops each of geranium, rose and lavender with 1 Tbs sweet almond oil.
- Apply neat as a perfume or in perfume blends; also use to scent pot pourris, linen, etc.
- Geranium makes a delightful, refreshing room fragrance – and repels insects.

GINGER *Zingiber officinale*

Ginger has been used as a traditional remedy and spice for thousands of years, especially in the East. It plays an important role in Chinese herbalism, where it is used principally for moist, cold, contracted conditions. It was known to the ancient Egyptians, and its use, principally as a culinary aid, was recorded in Greek and Roman times. It was regarded as a stimulant and tonic, having aphrodisiac properties. The Romans added it to wine to 'ginger it up'!

The flowers are traditionally worn by Hawaiian dancers, their *leis* being a combination of jasmine, carnation, gardenia and ginger lilies.

In Senegal and Fouta-Djalon, the women use pounded ginger root in the making of belts to arouse the dormant attention of their husbands.

> To the natives of the Pacific Islands of Dohu, ginger is sacred, and they use it in abundance in cooking, magic ritual and medicine. The witch doctor chews the root, and spits it on his patients' wounds and burns. The islanders believe it has remarkable healing effects.[31]

SCENT:
Exotic, fiery, fresh, penetrating, peppery, rich, slightly green, woody spicy. It blends well with cedarwood, coriander, frankincense, neroli, orange, patchouli and sandalwood.

KEY QUALITIES:
Aphrodisiac, cephalic, stimulating, tonic, warming.

CONTRA-INDICATIONS:
Ginger oil irritates the skin in concentration and may cause sensitization – use in low dilutions only.

It is also said that when there is a storm at sea, the fishermen chew the root and spit it into the water to make the waves abate!

It came to Europe via the 'spice route' in the Middle Ages and it was used to counter the plague, due to its anti-infectious properties. Crystallized ginger root is still popular in China and throughout Europe as a refreshing sweet and breath freshener.

In aromatherapy, the oil is considered to be a powerful nerve tonic, good for exhaustion and mental fatigue, and best used in combination with other oils. On a psychological level, it has a comforting, warming and uplifting effect on the emotions, and a stimulating effect on the mind.

APPLICATIONS & METHODS OF USE:

- Add 3 drops to the bath for nervous exhaustion, mental debility, frigidity, poor memory, impotence or migraine.
- For a stimulating aphrodisiac massage oil, blend 1 drop of ginger, 2 of jasmine and 3 of sandalwood in 1 Tbs sweet almond oil.
- Ginger is a stimulating, sensual room fragrance, but, again, is best blended with other oils.
- Add to perfume blends (in minute amounts), pot pourris, etc.

GRAPEFRUIT

– see Lemon

HOPS *Humulus lupulus*

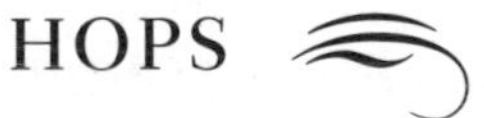

The name 'hop' is derived from the Anglo-Saxon word *hoppen*, meaning 'to climb', due to the plant's rambling nature. It has been used in both the East and West for thousands of years, both as a medicine and a form of nourishment. Traditionally, the Jewish captives in Babylon drank barley beer with hops, which kept them free of leprosy. Pliny records that the Romans cultivated hops as a garden plant and ate the young shoots as a vegetable.

Nowadays hops are best known for making beer in Britain, but that has not always been the case. Henry VI of England (1422–61) forbade the cultivation of this 'unwholesome weed', a prohibition continued by Henry VIII. It was not until 1524 that hops could be used for brewing beer in the Dutch style – before then, ale was generally made from malt in England.

During the seventeenth century, the hop plant became regarded as an important medicinal herb, and was commonly grown as a pot herb. It was

SCENT:
Rich, spicy, sweet, warm. Blends well with pine, nutmeg, citrus and spicy oils.

KEY QUALITIES:
Anaphrodisiac, hypnotic, narcotic, oestrogen properties, relaxing, sedative, soothing, soporific, tonic.

CONTRA-INDICATIONS:
Narcotic in large amounts – use in moderation. May cause sensitization in some individuals. Should be avoided by those suffering from depression, as hops depress the highest nervous functions.

prescribed for all types of nervous afflictions, including headaches, restlessness, anxiety, nervous exhaustion and delirium. In Europe and Asia a pillow stuffed with dried hops was a popular remedy for nervous tension, insomnia or nightmares. George III used a hop pillow to help him sleep when other sedative treatments failed to succeed.

It belongs to the same family as the well known drug cannabis and, like cannabis, has narcotic and hypnotic properties. It is also a powerful anaphrodisiac and produces a pronounced increase in the female oestrogen levels. A favourite herb of the gypsies, it was thought to cure 'uncontrolled sexual desires and a quarrelsome nature'.[32]

It is still employed in medical herbalism, principally as a general nerve tonic and sedative. It has been demonstrated that the aroma alone has the ability to have a calming effect on the body and mind.

APPLICATIONS & METHODS OF USE:

- To make a tea or tisane, take a dessertspoonful of dried flowers, add 1 pint (600 mls) of boiling water, let steep and add honey to taste. An excellent night-cap.
- Add 5–10 drops to a warm evening bath and inhale the vapours – good for nervous headaches, restlessness, irritability, anxiety, insomnia and nervous exhaustion.
- For a stress-relieving massage, hops are best used in combination with other relaxing oils, e.g. 3 drops each of hops and lavender or chamomile in 1 Tbs almond oil.
- Use the oil in a burner at night to help induce sleep or put a few drops on the pillow. Otherwise, stuff a pillow with dried hops (and lavender) in the traditional fashion.

HYSSOP 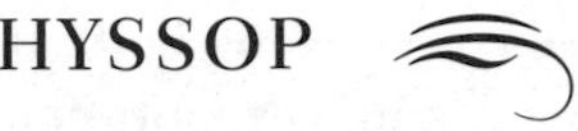 *Hyssopus officinalis*

The name 'hyssop' is derived from the Greek *hysoppus*, which in turn comes from the Hebrew *ezob*, meaning 'a good-scented herb'. This plant has an ancient medical reputation and was one of the bitter herbs used during the Passover ritual. In early times it was a symbol of baptism and the forgiveness of sins. It is thought to have been employed by both the Hebrews and the Egyptians to sweep out their temples and is mentioned several times in the Bible.

> Purge me with hyssop, and I shall be clean.[33]

However, it is possible, according to some scholars, that the plant referred to in the Bible was not *H. officinalis* but the caper plant or a form of marjoram, which are more commonly found in the Holy Land.

Whatever the case, hyssop has been held sacred as a plant of purification since early times. During pagan religious rituals it was sprayed on worshippers to cleanse them. It was valued by the ancient Greeks for similar reasons and Dioscorides referred to it as a 'holy herb' because it was used in the purification ceremonies in the form of incense. The Romans employed it both as a protection against plague and for its aphrodisiac effect in combination with ginger, thyme and pepper. It was also used for purifying and disinfecting the sick, notably lepers and leprous houses.

Although not indigenous to Britain, it was certainly known to the Cistercians, who favoured it as a bee plant, by the middle of the thirteenth century. It was planted in monastic gardens, and the religious extracted the oil as a flavouring for soups and

SCENT:
Herbaceous, slightly camphoraceous, sweet, warm. Blends with lavender, clary, geranium, rosemary and marjoram.

KEY QUALITIES:
Aphrodisiac, balancing, calming, cephalic, cleansing, mental stimulant, nervine, purifying, tonic, warming.

CONTRA-INDICATIONS:
Should be avoided by pregnant women, epileptics and children. The oil should be used in moderation.

sauces. During the fifteenth century it was also used as strewing herb. It was well known to the herbalists of the Middle Ages, and its reputation as a purifying herb has continued unchanged for centuries – it was used for the consecration of Westminster Abbey.

In herbal medicine it has been used principally for respiratory complaints but also as a general nerve tonic. It was once used in the treatment of anxiety, epilepsy and hysteria. As a tonic, it was also one of the ingredients of 'The herbal elixir of Grand-Chartreuse', together with lemon balm, angelica, cinnamon, saffron and mace.

On a psychological level, hyssop uplifts the spirit and gives the mind clarity and direction. Its warm scent helps calm emotional extremes and increases awareness.

APPLICATIONS & METHODS OF USE:

- Add 5–8 drops to the bath for anxiety, fatigue, depression, nervous tension and stress.
- The vaporized oil may be used to purify the environment and create clarity of mind. A good incense oil.
- Best blended with other oils for massage, e.g. 2 drops each of geranium, hyssop and lavender.

IMMORTELLE *Helichrysum angustifolia*

Closely related to the sunflower, this Mediterranean shrub has yellow, ball-like flowers which give off a curry-like scent when they are rubbed! Also known as everlasting and helichrysum, it was considered a valuable medicinal plant in earlier times. It is still used in the form of a decoction for headaches, migraine and liver ailments. Immortelle essential oil acts as a stimulant for the liver, gall bladder, spleen and pancreas as well as the whole endocrine system. It aids in the detoxification process, especially via the lymph glands.

In aromatherapy, it can be used to help cleanse the blood for people with allergies to environmental irritants or emotional imbalances, which manifest in conditions such as food rashes, eczema or psoriasis.

SCENT:
Floral green, gentle, rosy, slightly herbal, spicy, warm, woody.
It blends well with chamomile, cypress, lavender, neroli, rose and citrus oils.

KEY QUALITIES:
Calming, cleansing, comforting, drying, grounding, heating, inspirational, opening.

Immortelle oil has a strong psychological effect, emotionally warming and opening. It supports deep abdominal breathing and the scent has a relaxing, elevating effect on the mind. The scent of immortelle is also thought to increase dream activity and awareness, and to stimulate the right (intuitive) side of the brain. This makes it of use in meditation, active imagination and the creative arts. According to Patricia Davis, 'Helichrysum is said to induce feelings of compassion.'[34]

APPLICATIONS AND METHODS OF USE:

- Add 5–10 drops to the bath for all stress-related conditions.
- Use in massage blends, e.g. 2 drops each of immortelle, yarrow and chamomile in 1 Tbs base oil, to induce deep relaxation.
- As a vaporized oil, it may be used for meditation, yoga and visualization.

JASMINE *Jasminum officinale*

Native to Persia and Kashmir, jasmine was cultivated early in history. In Indian lore, Kama, the god of love, tips his arrows with jasmine blossoms to pierce the heart through the senses. Jasmine is known in India as 'Queen of the Night', because the scent is stronger during the hours of darkness. It was revered as a perfume of love in the Hindu and Muslim traditions. The *Medical Formulary* of Al-Kindi advises:

> Drug to excite intercourse: Throw in good oil of jasmine and asafoetida and leave it for some days. Then the male organ is oiled with that oil of jasmine at the time of intercourse. The woman is excited by its contact and she experiences a strong lust.[35]

The Arab poets sung its praises, and used it as symbol of divine and sexual aspiration and longing, as in the Sufi text *The Jasmine of the Fedeli D'Amore* by Ruzbehan Baqli of Shiraz. In China, jasmine was strewn on New Year's Day, hung from the eaves of house boats and as garlands and hair decorations. An account from 1777 tells of how clusters of unopened jasmine buds were picked at dawn, wrapped in damp cloth and sold at the market for use that same night when the flowers opened under the influence of moonlight and body heat, their romantic scent lingering until dawn.

The Chinese also used jasmine to cleanse the atmosphere surrounding the sick, and jasmine 'balls' were given to inebriated guests to clear the head of muzziness. It was also used in the treatment of nervous disorders, including insomnia and headaches, as a massage oil and a cosmetic.

In the West, jasmine reached a height of popularity in the late 1600s when the heady scents of orange, frangipani, neroli, tuberose and romane were in vogue. Later, Napoleon bought a large bottle of Spanish jasmine, as recorded by his perfumer Chardin, probably as a gift for Josephine. Louis XIV enjoyed jasmine-scented sheets. In European herbal medicine, jasmine was recommended for cold conditions, as 'it opens, warms and softens the nerves and tendons'.[36]

In aromatherapy, the oil is considered regulating and emotionally 'warming',

SCENT:
Exotic, exquisite, floral, long-lasting, rich, sweet, tea-like, warm.
Blends well with virtually everything, especially clary, cypress, neroli, orange, rose, sandalwood and ylang ylang.

KEY QUALITIES:
Anti-depressant, aphrodisiac, balancing, euphoric, intoxicating, tonic, uplifting, warming.

CONTRA-INDICATIONS:
Has been known to cause an allergic reaction in some individuals.

having a stimulating or sedative effect according to the individual need. The scent, according to Marcel Lavabre, is supremely sensual:

> Jasmine releases inhibition, liberates imagination, and develops exhilarating playfulness ... it has the power to transcend physical love and fully release both male and female sexual energy.[37]

Jasmine stimulates the brain to release 'encephaline', a neurotransmitter which acts as an analgesic and promotes a sense of well-being and even euphoria. The fragrance could be said to open the door of the emotions and penetrate to the soul of a person. It brings with it a feeling of confidence, optimism, warmth and trust. Psychological tension or fear is diminished, depression, sadness or confusion lifted. This is the basis for its aphrodisiac effect.

It is one of the most expensive but also one of the most vital ingredients in a wide range of perfumes. Most blends are enhanced by even a small percentage of jasmine. It is an especially useful addition to blends for psychosomatic disorders, such as skin problems or respiratory conditions triggered by underlying emotional causes.

N.B. There are many different varieties of jasmine – the so-called 'red jasmine' is frangipani, a Philippine plant.

APPLICATIONS & METHODS OF USE:

- Add 5–8 drops to the bath for depression, nervous exhaustion, apathy, indifference, listlessness, lack of confidence, grief, frigidity, PMT, menopausal problems, impotence, headaches, migraine and all stress-related conditions.
- An exquisite perfume in its own right – apply neat or in dilution.
- For an exotic sensual massage oil, blend 2 drops each of jasmine, ylang ylang and sandalwood and 1 of cardamom in 1 Tbs sweet almond oil.
- A reviving, uplifting and soothing room fragrance – use in an oil burner or add to pot pourris, etc.

JUNIPER *Juniperus communis*

There are over 40 species of juniper, including *J. phoenicea*, *J. communis* and *J. virginiana* (the oil of which is known as Virginian cedarwood). It was one of the early aromatics used in the ancient civilizations; remains of it have been found in a prehistoric Swiss lake dwelling. Juniper was also known to the ancient Egyptians and the oil was used to anoint the corpses in the mummification process. There are also other references to bodies being preserved with salt and juniper, as found in a fifth-century cemetery in Nubia and in a Coptic monastery at Thebes.

In Egypt, the wood and berries of juniper were used in the preparation of remedies and perfumes, and the berries were used together with cumin, moringa oil and frankincense to cure headaches.

In Roman times juniper was burned as an incense in the home and at funerals. Branches of juniper were also burned in ancient Greece to combat epidemics and more recently in French hospitals during the smallpox outbreak of 1870. It is still used as a purification incense by the Tibetans and as a medicine. The Native Americans burn dried sprigs of a form of juniper together with other herbs in ritual cleansing ceremonies.

In the Middle Ages it was considered a panacea for headaches, as well as being a potent diuretic and an antidote to plague. In Britain, it was thought that smoke from a juniper wood fire kept demons at bay and a spray of the berries was hung on the door on May Eve as protection against witchcraft. An infusion of the berries was thought to restore lost youth.

SCENT:
Balsamic, fresh, peppery, smoky, sweet, turpentine-like, woody.
It blends well with clary sage, cypress, elemi, galbanum, lavender, rosemary, vetiver, citrus and other woody oils.

KEY QUALITIES:
Antiseptic, aphrodisiac, clearing, protective, purifying, restorative, reviving, tonic (nerve).

CONTRA-INDICATIONS:
Avoid during pregnancy. Slightly irritating to the skin – use in moderation only. Not suitable for young children.

Culpeper claimed that it 'strengthened the brain' and the nerves, and was a good antiseptic.

> The cleansing properties of juniper work on the mental/emotional plane as well as the physical. It is a psychically purifying oil ... Juniper seems to clear 'waste' from the mind just as it does from the body.[38]

APPLICATIONS & METHODS OF USE:

- Add 5–8 drops to the bath for emotional exhaustion, weariness, feelings of uncleanness and mental stress.
- For a cleansing, restorative massage: blend 2 drops each of juniper, geranium and hyssop with 1 Tbs (12 ml) sweet almond oil.
- The vaporized oil makes an excellent purifying incense – effective on an environmental and psychological level. As a room fragrance, it clears the head, beneficial for intellectual fatigue, poor memory, tension headaches and mental confusion.
- A pleasing addition to perfume blends – especially men's fragrances.

LABDANUM  *Cistus ladaniferus*

Labdanum was one of the early aromatic substances of the ancient world. It is obtained from several species of the Cistus or rock rose family (*Cistinae*). It is listed in the Bible under the name 'Oncha' as an ingredient in the ancient temple incense of Moses. It was also used by the ancient Egyptians as an incense and for cosmetic purposes.

Especially abundant on the islands of Crete and Cyprus, labdanum resin was formerly collected by shepherds using a special instrument called a 'ladanisterion', by combing the sticky, balsamic substance from the fleeces of the sheep who brushed against it while grazing. This plant gives a characteristic smell to certain glades throughout Greece. It was most probably one of the aromatic materials sacred to Venus and burned on her fragrant altars on the island of Cyprus. The lumps of resin burn easily with a clear flame. Dioscorides recorded the ingredients for the so-called 'Royal Unguent', which included labdanum.

SCENT:
Amber, balsamic, dry, herbaceous, long-lasting, musky, rich, spicy, sweet, warm.
Blends well with cedarwood, clary sage, jasmine, lavender, lemon, neroli, woody and oriental oils.

KEY QUALITIES:
Anti-depressant, balancing, comforting, long-lasting, mild aphrodisiac, soothing, tonic, uplifting, warming.

CONTRA-INDICATIONS:
Avoid during pregnancy.

Since the Middle Ages in Europe, labdanum has been used in skin-care ointments for its healing, soothing properties – much like myrrh – and also as a base for perfumes. Its scent resembles ambergris, and it is extremely long-lasting and stable.

In aromatherapy, it is valued for its soothing, comforting warmth and mildly erotic qualities:

> Its essential oil conveys a warmth that deeply affects the soul. Rock rose is favoured for treating patients who feel, usually after a traumatic event, cold, empty or numb ... Rock rose incense aids meditation and centring as well as visualizing spiritual experiences and bringing them to consciousness.[39]

APPLICATIONS & METHODS OF USE:

- Add 5–10 drops to the bath to help counteract shock, grief, emotional coldness or frigidity.
- An excellent base for home perfume blends, warm, tenacious and rich.
- As an incense or room fragrance it is good for meditation and as a general relaxant; beneficial for stress-related complaints.
- Best blended with other oils for massage, e.g. 2 drops each of labdanum, rose and clary sage in 1 Tbs sweet almond oil.

LAVENDER *Lavendula angustifolia*

This fragrant herb has been cultivated since early times, and has been used for thousands of years. Its name, which derives from the Latin *lavare*, meaning 'to wash', refers to the Roman custom of scenting bath water with the aromatic leaves and flowers. In the East as well, especially in Turkey and Egypt, lavender has been used for centuries for perfuming the bath.

Lavender was mentioned by Dioscorides, Galen and Pliny, and it is known that the Romans traditionally used lavender in preparation for childbirth; the midwife also would trace a cross with the dried crushed leaves over hot coals, to fill the room with its fragrance during a birth.

Native to the Mediterranean region, lavender quickly spread throughout Europe and was especially popular in the medicinal monastery gardens of the thirteenth and fourteenth centuries. Lavender is still one the most popular garden flowers, though grown more for sentimental rather than practical reasons. It was one of the herbs dedicated to Hecate, the goddess of witches and sorcerers, but it was thought that a sprig of lavender could avert the 'evil eye'. It was strewn on the floors of houses and churches to keep off the plague, and on St Barnabas' Day chapels were decked with garlands of roses, box, woodruff and lavender.

Lavender water is one of the oldest English perfumes and Abbess Hildegarde, writing in the twelfth century, dedicated a whole chapter to the virtues of lavender – she recommended it for 'maintaining a pure character'.

In Elizabethan times ladies would sew sachets of lavender into their skirts, and the habit of using the flowers and leaves to scent linen and clothes and deter moths has retained its popularity even today. Lavender has also been used in pot pourris and for scenting leather and gloves – records from 1387 show that Charles VI of France was fond of lavender pillows. The very scent of lavender for many people still carries sentimental associations of times gone by ... childhood recollections of fresh linen in their grandmother's bedrooms and cuboards.

William Turner called it 'a comfort to the braine', and it was often used in the sick room to refresh and revive the fainting patient, sweeping away grief

SCENT:
Classic, floral, light, mellow, soft.
Blends well with bergamot, clary sage, geranium, lemon, neroli, orange, pine and rose.

KEY QUALITIES:
Anti-depressant, antiseptic, appeasing, balancing, calming, cephalic, cleansing, healing, insect repellent, purifying, relaxing, restorative, sedative, soothing.

and melancholy. Gerard said that the flowers helped to deter 'the panting and passion of the heart', and they had a reputation for keeping one chaste. Conversely, prostitutes once wore it extensively to advertise their trade and attract customers!

Matthiole, the sixteenth-century botanist, regarded lavender flowers as a most effective panacea for conditions such as epilepsy and apoplexy and for mental problems. Culpeper considered that lavender, governed by Mercury, was good for cold moist humours having a 'hot and subtle spirit'. Indeed, it has a long history of use as a nerve tonic, with a strengthening yet soothing effect. A sprig of lavender placed under the hat was used as a headache cure and to protect from sunstroke!

On a psychological level, the actions of lavender can be seen to 'mirror' many of its physical effects. It has a regulating effect, which is of great value to those who suffer from widely fluctuating mood states and feelings of emotional instability, including hysteria and manic depression.

Valnet recommends lavender as an evening bath oil for 'weak and delicate children', shock, tantrums, etc. Its fragrance certainly imparts a feeling of calm that allows one to let go of compulsions, irritation or anger. Lavender is being used increasingly in hospital wards today as a massage oil or airborne fragrance to help dispel anxiety, calm the mind and increase general feelings of well-being. It has also been used successfully in place of orthodox drugs to help patients sleep.

N.B. There are many varieties of lavender; the oil of aspic and lavandin have a more stimulating effect than that of *L. augustifolia* or *officinalis*, but are not of equal value for psychological or psychosomatic conditions.

Applications & Methods of Use:

- Add 5–10 drops to a warm evening bath to relieve insomnia, restlessness, anxiety, nervous tension, an over-active mind, sunstroke, hysteria, fear and other stress-related problems.
- For a restorative, healing massage, blend 2 drops each of lavender, rose and melissa in 1 Tbs sweet almond oil. Excellent for PMT,

menopausal problems, palpitations, grief, mood swings and depression.

- Put a few drops on a hanky and inhale, or apply neat to the temples to relieve headaches, giddiness, nausea, travel sickness, faintness or migraine.
- For a reviving room fragrance, blend lavender, lemon and bergamot together; good for mental debility, loss of memory and nervous weakness.
- To encourage relaxation or a restful night, use the vaporized oil in the bedroom, add to pot pourris, or put a few drops on the pillow or on pyjamas (excellent during pregnancy and for children). Sheets scented with lavender also induce sleep.
- Lavender is a traditional oil to vaporize in sick rooms, during childbirth or in the home to purify the air and to generally create a relaxed atmosphere.

LEMON  *Citrus limonum*

The lemon tree originated in South-East Asia, but during the second century AD it was introduced to Greece and then Italy, where it quickly adapted to the Mediterranean climate. Its name derives from the Arabic *limu* or *limun* and it is closely related to the lime, citron or cedrat fruit. It was known to the Greeks and Romans – Virgil called it the 'Median apple' because it came from Media near Persia. The ancients used the peel to perfume clothes and repel moths and other insects.

It was only later, during the seventeenth century in the West, that the medicinal qualities of lemon were recognized and used to counteract scurvy in the British Navy. According to the herbalist Lovell, its juice heals 'melancholy'.

Lemon conjures up images of freshness and cleanliness; its tangy, bright fragrance is refreshing and uplifting to the spirit. On a psychological level, the oil consequently has a clarifying quality, good for mental fatigue, listlessness or emotional confusion. The aroma alone stimulates the mind, increases the ability to memorize and improves intellectual performance. Brain research into the effects of fragrance has found that lemon oil primarily activates the centre of the hippocampus. Recent studies carried out in Japan show that the aroma of lemon increases concentration levels to a remarkable degree:

> They found that typing mistakes were reduced by 54% when lemon oil was disbursed in the room.[40]

The oil is particularly effective used in vaporized form for purifying the air and killing germs. It also stimulates the body's immune system and resistance levels.

It is being employed increasingly in hospitals today, not only as a disinfectant but also because it neutralizes unpleasant odours and disperses stale air. It has also been found to have a psychologically strengthening effect on usually depressed or fearful patients, especially in terminal wards.

SCENT:
Clean, fresh, lemony, light, penetrating.
Blends well with cedar, eucalyptus, fennel, juniper, lavender and pine.

KEY QUALITIES:
Antiseptic, cephalic, mental stimulant, purifying, refreshing, reviving, strengthening, tonic to the nervous and sympathetic nervous system.

CONTRA-INDICATIONS:
Photo-toxic – do not use lemon oil on skin exposed to direct sunlight or ultra-violet light. Irritant in concentration.

N.B. Grapefruit and lime oil have also been used for similar purposes. They all contain large amounts of the substance limonene and share similar therapeutic qualities.

APPLICATIONS & METHODS OF USE:

- Add up to 5 drops each of lemon and pine to a morning bath to overcome tiredness, sluggishness or a hangover.
- Use a few drops in a vaporizer in the study or office to aid concentration; or in a sick room to create a clean, fresh, uplifting atmosphere.
- For a stimulating, restorative massage, combine 2 drops each of lemon, pine and juniper in 1 Tbs sweet almond oil.

- Fresh lemon juice can also help overcome symptoms of PMT – for a week prior to menstruation, drink a hot lemon drink first thing in the morning and last thing at night.

LIME

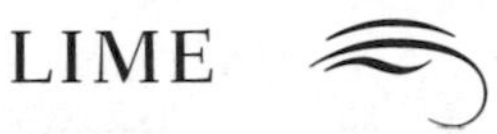

– see Lemon

LINDEN *Tilia vulgaris*

In old herbals the lime tree was called lyne, linc, tillet, till tree or tilia, and the fragrant feathery flowers were known as linnflowers or linden. The linden or lime tree was the ancient emblem of Germanic countries, and to this day they are still commonly found in villages and beside roads throughout the region. Although the flowers are highly scented they are virtually invisible, because they are hidden by the leaves which are of the same colour.

The Romans were familiar with the benefits of linden, and they are mentioned by Pliny and other writers. It is also known to have been planted in the medicinal gardens of ancient Egypt. It was well known as a bee plant, and honey from the flowers is widely regarded as of the best flavour.

According to Culpeper it is governed by Jupiter, and the flowers are 'a good cephalic and nervine, excellent for apoplexy, epilepsy, vertigo and palpitation of the heart'.[41]

In herbal medicine, linden is recommended for migraine, hypertension, hysteria, headaches, dizziness and for any disorder involving nervous stress or tension – 'pains in the head of a cold cause'.

In both England and France it has been traditionally used for palpitations, nervous dyspepsia and nervous weakness. Large amounts of lime flowers were collected during the Second World War for medical use. Linden tea, known as *tilleul*, is still a popular drink on the Continent, especially in France, where it is used to soothe the nerves and to help induce sleep. It is especially recommended for over-excited or restless

SCENT:
Green, hay-like, honey, soft. It blends well with bergamot, chamomile, immortelle and mimosa.

KEY QUALITIES:
Calming, cleansing, drying, sedating, soothing, uplifting, warming.

CONTRA-INDICATIONS:
Frequently subject to adulteration.

children. The tea is also a gentle tonic, good for nervous debility and as a blood purifier.

In aromatherapy, the oil is beneficial for all types of nervous afflictions – excellent for stress-related conditions. As a tonic, it is also beneficial for depression and listlessness.

APPLICATIONS & METHODS OF USE:

- Add 5 –10 drops to a warm bath to soothe nervous irritability, anxiety or restlessness and induce restful sleep.
- For a traditional relaxing tea, add a tablespoon of dried leaves to ½ litre of boiling water, let steep and add honey to taste. A good after-dinner drink or night-cap. Sheets scented with linden smell sweet and fragrant and help induce restful sleep.
- The vaporized oil soothes the nerves, calms the mind and uplifts the spirits – a good remedy for headaches and migraine.
- A massage oil, good for all stress-related conditions, can be made by mixing 5 drops of linden with 1 Tbs sweet almond oil.
- The dried leaves or oil can be added to pot pourris.

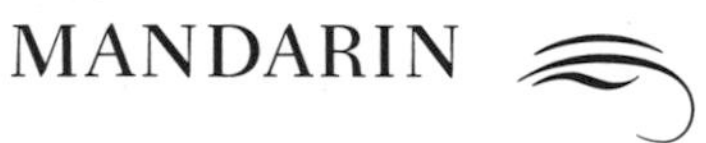

MANDARIN

see Orange

MARJORAM, SWEET 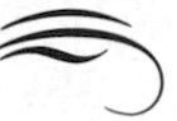 *Oreganum majorana*

There are many different varieties of this herb apart from sweet marjoram, notably wild marjoram (*Origanum vulgare*), pot marjoram (*M. onites*) and Spanish marjoram (*Thymus mastichina*). The botanical name *oreganum* derives from the Greek, meaning 'joy of the mountain'. Pot marjoram was grown by the ancient Egyptians. They called it 'suampsuchum' and used it in perfumes, unguents and medicines from the earliest times. The plant was considered sacred to Osiris in Egypt, and to Shiva and Vishnu in India.

The Greeks used wild marjoram extensively as a remedy and planted it on graves, believing that it would help the dead to sleep in peace. Among the Greeks and Romans alike it was a symbol of love and honour, and it was the custom to crown young married couples with marjoram. In myth, it was associated with Aphrodite and Venus.

Dioscorides himself made a pomade called 'amaricimum' with marjoram for nervous disorders, while Theophrastus wrote an interesting account of its use in perfumery, since it had the lasting scent that women required.

In England sweet marjoram was cultivated by monks in their herbariums from the thirteenth century onward. Infusions of the powdered tops were taken for nervous complaints and marjoram was widely thought of as an antidote to poison. Bunches were hung up in the dairy or placed between pails of milk to keep it fresh, especially during warm or stormy weather. During the Tudor period it was used as a strewing herb and continued to be used in this way up to the end of the seventeenth century. Even the smell of it was thought to keep one in good health and it was one of Elizabeth I's favourite scents. It was used, according to the London herbalist Parkinson, 'to please the outward senses in nosegaies', as well as in 'sweete powders', 'sweete bags' and 'sweete washing waters'. Powdered marjoram was also used to scent winding sheets and was thought to comfort the bereaved as well as the dead! According to Culpeper:

SCENT:
Camphoraceous, herbaceous, nutty, penetrating, spicy, warm, woody.
It blends well with bergamot, cedarwood, chamomile, cypress, eucalyptus, lavender and rosemary.

KEY QUALITIES:
Analgesic, anaphrodisiac, antiseptic, cephalic, comforting, nervine, restorative, sedative, warming.

CONTRA-INDICATIONS:
Avoid during pregnancy; stupefying in large doses.

> It is an herb of Mercury and under Aries, and is an excellent remedy for the brain and other parts of the body. Our Common Sweet marjoram is warming and comforting in cold diseases of the head...[42]

The fresh leaves were added to the bath as a tonic, while the oil was used for insomnia, nausea and headaches. In 1720, Monsieur Chomel, head of the Academy of Medicine in France, recommended powdered marjoram to be taken like snuff as an inhalation to fortify the brain and reduce fatigue. In 1876, F. J. Cazin prescribed marjoram for all types of nervous disorders, including apoplexy, paralysis, dizziness, epilepsy and loss of memory. The folk herbalist Juliette de Baïracli Levy uses it for morning sickness, shaky nerves, fears, depression, nightmares and bed-wetting.

In aromatherapy, it is employed for its antiseptic, cephalic, sedative and nervine properties. On a psychological level, its warm and penetrating odour is relaxing, soothing and fortifying to the mind. It is also considered useful for those suffering from grief or loneliness, but it should not be over-used since it can have a deadening effect on the emotions. This is most probably the basis for its use as an anaphrodisiac by religious institutions in the past.

APPLICATIONS & METHODS OF USE:

- An excellent sedative oil; add 5–10 drops to an evening bath to relieve all types of stress – headache, hypertension, migraine, insomnia, PMT, anxiety, mental fatigue/strain, overwork, etc.
- For a relaxing yet restorative massage, mix 6 drops of marjoram with 1 Tbs sweet almond oil, rub clockwise into the soles of the feet, the

solar plexus and along the spine. Good for mental or nervous debility and stress.

- The vaporized oil is clearing and purifying, both on a physical and mental level.

MELISSA *Melissa officinalis*

Commonly known as 'lemon balm' or 'heart's delight', this herb has an ancient healing reputation. The name derives from the Greek nymph Melissa, protectress of the bees, because they find its scent irresistible. Theophrastus and Dioscorides considered it a potent sedative; Avicenna recommended it for its cheering effect; other Moslem and Arab writers prescribed it for melancholy and heart complaints. It was introduced into northern Europe by the Romans, who used it as a relaxant and added it to their bath water. The alchemist Paracelsus called it 'The Elixir of Life' for he believed that its use guaranteed long life.

An entry in the *London Dispensary* (1696) reads:

> An essence of Balm drunk every morning will renew youth, strengthen the brain, relieve languishing nature, and prevent baldness.[43]

It is said that the Welsh Prince Llewelyn lived to the age of 108 by following this simple habit, while John Hussey of Sydenham, who lived to 116, breakfasted for 50 years on balm tea with honey.

It was also known as the 'scholar's herb'. Thomas Coghan, a sixteenth-century Oxford don, recommended that the tea was drunk daily by his students to help clear the head, increase understanding and sharpen the memory. According to Culpeper, it is under Jupiter and in the sign of Cancer. He says that it 'driveth away all troublesome cares and thoughts out of the mind'. Gerarde also commented that 'it maketh the heart merry and joyful and strengtheneth the vitall spirits'.

In France, melissa was *the* ingredient of the famous 'Carmelite water', an early type of eau de cologne distilled in Paris since 1611 by monks – it was also used for nervous headaches and neuralgic affections. Balm was also used as a strewing herb and grown in every country garden.

The dried leaves retain their scent for a long time, so it made a good addition to herb pillows, pot pourris, etc. It can also be used to deter moths from clothes and linen. 'Balm Oil' is still a favourite scent throughout the Middle East, especially among the Arabs. The oil contains large amounts of citral and citronellol, substances which have been found to have a direct sedative effect on the nervous system.

More recently, the psychological effects of melissa have been subjected to scientific research:

> The sedative effects of 'spirit of Melissa' have been demonstrated in the treatment of psychiatric disorders such as vegetative dystonia; significant improvement in the symptoms (restlessness, excitability, palpitations and headache) was obtained.[44]

In aromatherapy, melissa oil is used as a tonic and sedative for the nervous system – valuable for all types of stress-related conditions. However, it is on an emotional level that melissa is outstanding, having traditionally been used as a tonic for the heart and a remedy for the 'distressed spirit'. The oil acts on the vital centre and helps balance delicate or vacillating emotions. Patricia Davis writes:

> It has long been known for its ability to bring comfort to the bereaved ... I have also found Melissa a great help and comfort to those who know that they are dying, as well as their friends and relatives.[45]

N.B. Lemon verbena (*Aloysia triphylla*) shares similar properties, but the essential oil is difficult to get hold of in unadulterated form.

SCENT:
Fresh, green, herbaceous, honey sweet, lemony, light. It blends well with geranium, lavender, myrtle, neroli and rose.

KEY QUALITIES:
Appeasing, calming, comforting, heart tonic, protecting, regulating, revitalizing, sedative, soothing, strengthening, uplifting.

CONTRA-INDICATIONS:
Use in low dilutions only (not above 1 per cent) as it can cause skin irritation in concentration and is narcotic in large doses, causing headaches. True melissa is costly: beware of adulteration!

APPLICATIONS & METHODS OF USE:

- For a soothing evening bath, add up to 5 drops to the bath water and inhale the fragrance. Good for insomnia, nervous tension, anxiety, depression, nervous exhaustion, nightmares and stress.
- A melissa massage is a comforting experience in itself, beneficial for all states of emotional imbalance – add 3 drops of melissa to 1 Tbs almond oil. Good for PMT, menopausal symptoms, eczema, palpitations, grief, shock, anger, depression and post-natal depression.
- The vaporized oil makes a delightful fresh, lemony room fragrance and a good insect repellent.
- Inhaling the odour, by putting a few drops on a hanky, is also good for all types of complaint with a nervous origin, such as asthma, headaches, migraine and faintness.
- Lemon balm makes an excellent uplifting and rejuvenating tea. Add a handful of fresh leaves or a dessertspoonful of dried leaves to a pint (600 ml) of boiling water, steep and add honey to taste.
- Add the dried leaves or a few drops of essential oil to pot pourris, or to scent sheets, clothes, linen, etc. – it helps deter moths.

MINT – PEPPERMINT 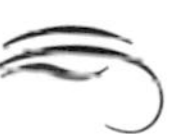 *Mentha piperita*

There are many different varieties of mint, but those which have enjoyed the longest tradition usage are probably peppermint and spearmint *(M. spicata)*.

Peppermint was cultivated by the ancient Egyptians – remains of the dried leaves from a bouquet have been found in a tomb dating from about 300 BC. Dioscorides also mentions that mint was an ingredient of the famous Egyptian perfume and remedy 'Kyphi'.

Mint has been used extensively in the East as a tonic for thousands of years. Legend says that the priest Enzan brought peppermint plants from China to Japan for cultivation in about AD 200. The Bible mentions mint being used as a tithe or tribute, which shows that it was also valued throughout the Middle East. The Jews once strewed the floors of their synagogues with mint so that its clean, purifying perfume scented the place as they entered for worship.

Mint was a favourite of the Greeks and Romans, who used crowns of peppermint to adorn themselves on festive occasions. It was also worn by brides. Its name derives from the Latin *mente*, meaning 'thought', because the Romans considered it a tonic for the brain. In later times, mint was dedicated to the Virgin Mary. According to Greek myth, it is named after Mintha, a lover of Pluto whom Persephone, in a fit of rage, ground into the earth, from whence a herb sprung up that has since borne her name. They believed that it 'stirred the passions' and forbade its use to soldiers in time of war in case it diverted their attentions! Indeed, both peppermint and spearmint stimulate the whole metabolism, especially the heart and circulation, and also strengthen the nerves. The Greeks used mint to scent their bath water and as a general restorative in the same way as smelling salts. They used lemon mint for making perfumes and in powdered form sprinkled it in their bedding so as to scent the whole body. Pliny wrote, 'The very smell of mint restores and revives the spirit just as its taste excites the appetite.'

SCENT:
Bright, clean, fresh, minty, penetrating.
It blends well with eucalyptus, lavender, lemon and rosemary.

KEY QUALITIES:
Antiseptic, aphrodisiac, cephalic, nerve tonic, refreshing, restorative, stimulant (mental).

CONTRA-INDICATIONS:
Do not use the oil in combination with homeopathic remedies. Used in strong doses it can inhibit sleep. In concentration it brings to the skin a burning or tingling sensation – use in dilution only.

During the Middle Ages, mint was a favourite strewing herb, for, according to Gerard, 'The smelle rejoiceth the heart of man.' He also considered it 'a good Posie for students oft to smell', and especially beneficial for those of weak constitution. According to Culpeper, it is a herb of Venus and 'being smelled into, it is comfortable for the head and memory ... '[46]

In herbal medicine, it has been used for palpitations of the heart, hysteria and other nervous disorders. It is also an effective pain-killer, which can be helpful for many nervous complaints especially headaches and migraine. Peppermint is one of the oils described as 'cephalic', that is, it stimulates the mind and aids clear thinking. Physically, it helps clear congestion. Like basil and lemon, it stimulates the central hippocampus of the brain, encouraging concentration.

Mint soothes as well as excites. The oil has a warming, comforting quality when it is applied to the skin, for although it is described as cooling, it stimulates the cold-perceiving nerves and thus brings a sensation of warmth.

It has a long-standing reputation as an aphrodisiac. Once esteemed as a cure for frigidity in both sexes, even today it is used as a tonic for bulls and stallions when their sexual powers are waning. The Arabs still drink mint tea frequently to ensure virility.

N.B. Spearmint is milder then peppermint, making it more suitable for children.

APPLICATIONS & METHODS OF USE:

- Add 3 drops to bath water for a refreshing and reviving morning bath. It is also beneficial for depression, convalescence, nervous exhaustion, mental fatigue, impotence, frigidity and stress-related conditions.
  N.B. Do not use more than 3 drops of peppermint in the bath, or more than 5 drops of spearmint, due to possible irritation.
- Peppermint oil makes a good addition to a restorative massage oil blend, used in combination with other oils of similar properties such as basil or rosemary, e.g. 2 drops each of peppermint, basil and rosemary in 1 Tbs sweet almond oil.
- A few drops of oil on a hanky or in a vaporizer can be inhaled to help clear the head of congestion, revive the spirit and improve concentration. The vaporized oil is also very useful for respiratory conditions of nervous origin, notably asthma. Its strong penetrating, slightly camphoraceous odour can also can help overcome faintness, dizziness or shock.
- An excellent headache or migraine remedy is to make a compress using a flannel or cloth dipped in a small bowl of iced water which

contains a few drops of peppermint oil. Squeeze out the cloth and lay this across the forehead, renewing frequently.

- A good tonic to fortify the nerves, increase sexual prowess or simply as a quick pick-me-up tea can be made by putting a few freshly chopped leaves (or a dessertspoonful of dried herb) in a pint (600 ml) of boiling water, leaving to stand for 5 minutes, then sipping slowly (sweeten with honey if desired).
- As a room fragrance or added to pot pourris peppermint has a cleansing, purifying quality. It is one of the best oils for overcoming the smell of cigarette smoke and is also a good insect repellent.

MYRRH *Commiphora myrrha*

Myrrh has been used for over 3,700 years; it was one of the first substances found to provide a powerful and lasting scent. The name derives from the Arabic *murr*, meaning 'bitter'. Myrrh was highly esteemed as a perfume, incense and remedy throughout the Near East and entire Mediterranean region. The Vedas and the Koran mention numerous uses of myrrh in religious ceremonies and perfumes and as a healing agent.

In Egypt's Heliopolis, city of the sun god Ra, incense was burned three times a day to mark the stations of the sun's journey and myrrh or 'punt' was used as high noon. It was also used by the Egyptians in fumigants, cosmetics and healing ointments including the famous 'Kyphi', a perfume and remedy combined. The vapours were prescribed for hayfever, and during mummification the stomach of the corpse was stuffed with myrrh and cassia before being sewn up.

In many Eastern countries where water was scarce, a lump of myrrh was hung around the neck where the body heat caused the fragrance to diffuse as a purifying agent.

Myrrh is mentioned in the Bible, where it is called 'bdellium', and together with frankincense was given to the Christ child by the Magi at his birth. It is included in the Jews' 'holy oil' and referred to in the 'Song of Solomon'. Esther and other Hebrew women used myrrh as part of their purification rituals that were carried out throughout the year. Myrrh was used for half the period. Moses took myrrh with him from Egypt so the Children of Israel could continue their form of worship. In the New Testament, Nicodemus ordered 100 lb of myrrh and aloe to anoint the body of Jesus, as was the custom of the time. The Hebrews mixed myrrh with their wine to raise their state of consciousness before participating in religious ceremonies. The same mixture was also given to criminals before their execution to help ease their suffering.

SCENT:
Balsamic, bitter, long-lasting, resinous, rich, spicy.
It blends well with cypress, frankincense, geranium, juniper, lavender, mandarin, mint, patchouli, pine, sandalwood, thyme and spicy oils.

KEY QUALITIES:
Healing, purifying, restorative, revitalizing, sedative (nerve), soothing, uplifting,

CONTRA-INDICATIONS:
Do not use during pregnancy.

The Greeks valued myrrh, which they called *balsamodendron*. According to Greek legend, myrrh originated from the tears of Myrrha, daughter of the King of Cyprus, who was transformed into the aromatic shrub. It was the main ingredient of 'Megalion', the famous unguent and perfume, which was warming and mollifying. The Greeks also combined it with red-flowered lilies in the fragrant ointment 'Susinum' – still popular in Rome around 450 BC. Indeed, it is mentioned by most of the ancient Greek and Roman writers, including Herodotus, Theophrastus, Dioscorides and Pliny, who all praised its powerful antiseptic qualities and included it in many healing salves.

In traditional Tibetan medicine, myrrh resin is still included in a recipe for relieving stress and nervous disorders. Either the medicated fumes are inhaled or it is employed as a massage oil.

The Chinese physician Li Shih-Chen says:

> It is regarded as an alterative [regulating agent] and sedative, and, as formerly in the West, is used in the treatment of wounds and ulcers ... also in the treatment of a disease resembling hysterical mania.[47]

In the West myrrh has traditionally been considered to have an opening, heating, drying nature, which stimulates the mind and fortifies the nerves, being especially good for those suffering from nervous weakness or debility. Like many aromatics, it combines a soothing, mollifying and restorative effect on the nerves with an uplifting and rejuvenating effect on the mind and spirit.

In aromatherapy it is used mainly for skin care, but is also valued for its psychological effect. According to Patricia Davis:

> Myrrh is particularly valuable for people who feel stuck emotionally or spiritually and want to move forward in their lives.[48]

APPLICATIONS & METHODS OF USE:

- This oil makes a excellent 'burning perfume' or incense. The vaporized oil has a purifying, uplifting and healing quality which is conducive to meditation, prayer, yoga, etc. The vaporized oil also has a warming, soothing and antiseptic effect which is valuable for respiratory conditions of nervous origin such as asthma and hayfever.
- Myrrh blends well with rose and sandalwood for a comforting, stress-relieving bath – add 3 drops of each oil to the bath water and relax.
- Use in combination with other oils in massage oil blends for convalescence, nervous exhaustion, mental fatigue and general debility, e.g. 2 drops each of myrrh, sandalwood and rose in 1 Tbs carrier oil.
- The oil makes an excellent addition to home perfume blends, pot pourris or pomanders due to its excellent long-lasting, tenacious and fixative properties.

MYRTLE 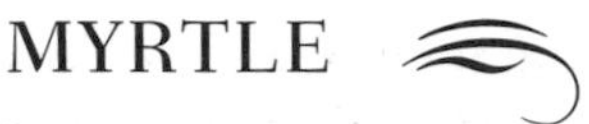 *Myrtus communis*

This attractive evergreen shrub from the Mediterranean has been described in myth and legend for centuries. In Egypt the leaves were used along with other aromatics for fumigation, primarily for respiratory and nervous afflictions. Pliny informs us that the myrtle with most powerful, pungent scent grew in Egypt. Dioscorides describes how the leaves were steeped in olive oil to make a highly fragrant oil for anointing the body. The leaves, berries and oil were in fact used in numerous ancient medicines.

According to myth, the goddess Aphrodite (or Venus) sought refuge beneath a myrtle bush when she first emerged naked from the sea. Since then myrtle has stood for chaste beauty, purity and love. Yet the goddess of love is also associated with death. Youth and innocence must pass away inevitably ... still her beauty intimates that there must be a life after death, just as the spirit or soul's purity remains eternal.

According to Greek and Roman folklore, myrtle tea, drunk at least once every three days preserves love and youth. In love affairs, the lover and the beloved would imbibe the drink together to ensure mutual devotion. Some women in the south of France still drink myrtle tea to help retain their beauty. It was also traditional in southern France to plant a myrtle bush by the house as protection against the evil eye. However, this was only said to be effective if carried out by a woman.

In Biblical times, Jewish women wore garlands of myrtle at their wedding as a symbol of conjugal love and to bring them luck. An ancient wreath of myrtle leaves and flowers has been discovered. Many brides today still wear myrtle as a symbol of innocence and virginity. The leaves and flowers were a major ingredient of the so-called 'angel's lotion', a

SCENT:
Balsamic, camphoraceous, clear, diffusive, floral, fresh, spicy, sporty.
It blends well with bay, bergamot, clary sage, lavender, lemon, neroli, rosemary and spicy oils.

KEY QUALITIES:
Antiseptic, aphrodisiac, clarifying, cleansing, mildly stimulating, refreshing, tonic (nerve), uplifting.

sixteenth-century refreshing skin-care lotion and deodorant.

In Italy and Greece, myrtle has long been a popular remedy for children's respiratory ailments, because of its antiseptic yet mild action. According to Lovell, 'The oile of myrtle is good in commotion of the brain ... it strengthens the brain and nerves.'[49] The folk usage and many of the properties mentioned in the old medical texts were later confirmed by the twentieth-century French researcher M. Linarix in a thorough scientific investigation, which he concluded by saying that myrtle was 'the best tolerated of all the balsamic oils'.[50]

In aromatherapy, it is valued primarily as an astringent, antiseptic skin-care agent and as a mild alternative to eucalyptus or other camphoraceous oils, such as cajeput or niaouli. Myrtle's psychological effect is reflected in its mythic associations, for its scent has a light, pure, refreshing quality – a youthful charm.

> Myrtle is helpful for people whose body seems draped in a grey, brown veil from smoking, drug abuse, or emotions like anger, greed, envy or fear. In such cases myrtle helps cleanse the person's delicate inner being to dissolve disharmony ... The oil acts as a friend in life transitions.[51]

N.B. Not to be confused with calamus oil (*Acorus calamus*), also known as 'sweet myrtle'.

Applications & Methods of Use:

- Add 5–10 drops to the bath for a purifying, refreshing effect. Good for breaking old negative habit patterns.
- The vaporized oil has a fresh, clean fragrance – it seems to purify both the environment and the psyche. An excellent oil to burn in a room for children's respiratory complaints, especially those of nervous origin.
- Put a few drops on a hanky for use throughout the day as a reviving deodorant.
- Also good in pot pourris and for keeping insects at bay.

NARCISSUS — *Narcissus poeticus*

The name probably derives from the Greek word *narkao*, meaning 'to numb', or *narce*, meaning 'torpor or lethargy', for, according to Pliny, the herbaceous narcissus can produce a heavy, dull sensation in the head. The legend of the handsome Greek youth who fell in love with his own image and was changed into a narcissus flower also tells us something about its intoxicating quality. The Greeks saw it as a portent of death and planted it near their graveyards. The Arabians considered it an aphrodisiac, and in India the oil is applied to the body before prayer in temples along with rose, sandalwood and jasmine.

> Narcissus may well be the stuff that dreams are made of, inspirational or intoxicating, imaginative or hallucinogenic … the mesmerising quality of Narcissus seems to afford it a place within the spiritual and carnal worlds.[52]

In France the flowers were once used for their antispasmodic qualities; the plant was said to be helpful for hysteria and epilepsy. However, it has been noted that the scent of the flowers can be overpowering if they are present in any quantity in a closed room, and can even cause headaches or nausea.

In aromatherapy, narcissus may be used in moderation for its sedating yet inspirational effects. Earthy and hypnotic, it can be deeply relaxing, yet full of sensuality.

N.B. There are several varieties of narcissus, including *N. jonquilla*, *N. pseudonarcissus* and *N. bulbocodium*.

APPLICATIONS & METHODS OF USE:

- Use in small quantities in exotic personal perfumes and other blends.
- The vaporized oil may be of value in creative work, for melting artistic blocks.

SCENT:
Sweet, green, herbaceous, heavy floral undertone. It blends well with clove, sandalwood, ylang ylang and other floral fragrances.

KEY QUALITIES:
Aphrodisiac, hallucinogenic, hypnotic, inspirational, intoxicating, narcotic, sedating.

CONTRA-INDICATIONS:
Use in moderation.

NEROLI BIGARADIA  *Citrus aurantium var. amara*

The soft floral fragrance of neroli oil, distilled from the blossoms of the bitter orange tree, was not discovered until the sixteenth century, although oranges had been known from the first century AD. Neroli was named after Anna Maria de la Tremoille, Princess of Neroli in Italy, who loved its delicate fragrance and used it to scent her bath water and perfume her gloves, scarves, shawls, etc.

Neroli was also highly valued for its therapeutic qualities by the people of Venice, who used it to combat the plague and fever, and drank it as a tea to help overcome nervous afflictions. Orange-flower water became popular all over Europe during the early eighteenth century and was rubbed onto the body twice a day. It still remains one of the most popular toilet waters.

At one time neroli was used a great deal by the prostitutes of Madrid and the scent became associated with that profession. Later, the white scented blossoms came to symbolize purity and, like myrtle, were traditionally used in bridal wreaths and bouquets. Since neroli also has the reputation for being an aphrodisiac, the profane and sacred aspects of love are here closely intermingled.

On the Continent, an infusion of the dried flowers is still used as a mild tonic for the nervous system and as a blood cleanser. Neroli oil has a soothing, supportive action on the heart. It is especially useful for anxious, fearful types who worry unnecessarily. Neroli oil is also a valuable remedy for shock or for disorders caused by a trauma, causing a strain on the heart.

The effect of neroli oil on the mind is soothing, tranquillizing and slightly hypnotic. This makes it a particularly useful remedy for all types of stress-related complaints:

> I find that by far the most important uses of Neroli are in helping with problems of emotional origin. It is especially valuable for states of anxiety.[53]

The scent of neroli has a pure uplifting quality which also makes it beneficial for depression and mental lethargy. It seems to have the ability to touch the very soul or essence of a person, bringing renewal and hope. It is also thought by some to enhance the process of creativity.

N.B. Petitgrain oil, which is extracted from the leaves of the orange tree, has very similar properties to neroli, though not as pronounced, being a sedative, relaxant, tranquillizer and cardiac tonic.

SCENT:
Delicate, floral, pervasive, rich, soft, sweet, warm.
It blends well with virtually all oils, notably chamomile, clary sage, geranium, jasmine, lavender, rose, ylang ylang and other citrus oils.

KEY QUALITIES:
Anti-depressant, aphrodisiac, hypnotic, restorative, sedative, soothing, tonic, uplifting.

APPLICATIONS & METHODS OF USE:

- Add 4–8 drops to the bath before retiring to help induce a restful sleep and banish anxiety, nervous tension or restlessness. Taking regular neroli baths in the week before menstruation also helps relieve PMT.
- Mix 3 drops of neroli oil with one tsp sweet almond oil and massage clockwise into the solar plexus, chest and the nape of the neck to help soothe palpitations, emotional shock or grief. Neroli is one of the best oils for those prone to depression.
- The vaporized oil has a purifying, uplifting yet relaxing quality, and is excellent as a bedroom fragrance (especially considering its aphrodisiac qualities), but also conducive to meditation, prayer, etc.
- Neroli is exquisite worn simply as a perfume. It can also be used to scent clothes, gloves, scarves or linen in traditional fashion – orange-blossom scented gloves were known as guanti de neroli.
- A cup of orange-blossom tea drunk in the evening is a good nerve restorative, and excellent for those who lead a hectic life and find it difficult to relax or sleep.
- Since neroli is a very safe oil, it can be used with great benefit during pregnancy and labour to create a feeling of calmness and ease. Two to five drops may also be added to children's baths to help overcome restlessness or excitability.

NUTMEG *Myristica fragrans*

First mentioned in the fifth century, nutmeg was introduced to the Occident by Arabian traders. In Europe during the Middle Ages, it was considered one of the most valuable commodities from the Orient, due to its many therapeutic and culinary uses, and it was used in a wide variety of unguents, elixirs and balms. Portugal monopolized the trade until 1605, when the Dutch took over. Prices were kept high by the destruction of trees outside the plantations; huge piles of the spice were even burned to ensure its value. In 1704, Pulligny wrote more than 800 pages on the virtues of nutmeg.

According to the Doctrine of Signatures, nutmeg was used as a remedy for all mental ailments, due to its resemblance to the human brain. It was well known as a narcotic and the oil was commonly used as an opiate. The potentially poisonous and hallucinogenic effects of nutmeg were first recorded in Europe by Lobelius in 1579. It is said that the scent of the Nutmeg Islands is so powerful that birds of paradise become intoxicated. In southern India, nutmeg mixed with betel and snuff is taken as a euphoric; in certain parts of Indonesia it is powdered down and snuffed on its own.

During the eighteenth century, a little silver nutmeg grater was often carried by the woman of the house, to make nutmeg tea for a night-cap. Nutmeg brandy was also made as a soporific:

> 3 ozs (85 g) grated nutmeg were put into a bottle of brandy, corked, and shaken once every day for a fortnight. After being left to settle, the liquid was poured off without disturbing the sediment. Ten drops in a glass of hot milk or water was the usual dose.[54]

It was also used a mild pain-killer and had the reputation of being a potent aphrodisiac. Its slightly euphoric effects have been associated with clairvoyance and divination. The scent alone has a warming, comforting and elevating effect on the mind.

In herbal medicine nutmeg is considered a powerful tonic and stimulant of the heart and circulation. In 1722 Joseph Miller wrote of the seeds:

> They are heating and drying … comfort the head and nerves, cure palpitation of the heart and prevent swooning, and are of service against vapours.[55]

In Tibetan medicine it is considered especially good for palpitations, anxiety, restlessness, agitation, depression and other neurotic symptoms. Like cinnamon, it is considered especially good for those with a *rlung* type of temperament, i.e. nervous, worried, talkative people who think too much and sleep too little. It is applied either in a massage oil or as a fumigant.

N.B. Oil of mace has similar properties but is more toxic and should be avoided for therapeutic use.

SCENT:
Oriental, rich, sensual, spicy, sweet, warm.
It blends well with bay, clary sage, geranium, orange, rosemary, oriental and spicy oils.

KEY QUALITIES:
Analgesic, aphrodisiac, calming, cephalic, comforting, elevating, euphoric, narcotic, soothing, tonic (nerve and heart).

CONTRA-INDICATIONS:
Stupefying and toxic in high doses – can cause delirium, hallucinations or fainting. Skin irritant in concentration. Avoid during pregnancy. Use with care, in moderation. Not suitable for young children.

APPLICATIONS & METHODS OF USE:

- Add 3 drops (no more) to an evening bath to help combat frigidity, nervous tension or insomnia.
- Use the vaporized oil in a burner or apply a few drops to a hanky for feelings of anxiety, depression, nervous weakness or mental fatigue. As a room fragrance it creates a warm, euphoric atmosphere.
- It blends well with orange and cinnamon leaf for a tonic yet soothing massage oil. Mix 3 drops each of nutmeg, cinnamon and orange with 1 Tbs sweet almond oil and massage slowly into the solar plexus in a clockwise direction for nervous dyspepsia, agitation and other symptoms of stress.
- A soothing night-cap can be made by sprinkling a little grated or powdered nutmeg on the top of a hot milk drink at bedtime.

ORANGE *Citrus aurantium*

The orange tree originated in eastern Asia, but the forebear of all today's varieties of orange was probably the bitter or Seville orange. It was first brought to the Mediterranean region by the Arabs in the first century AD, but it was not until the eighth century that oranges became commonly established in Spain.

The therapeutic value of oranges was first mentioned in Arab and Chinese herbals. By the tenth century in Europe, oranges were recommended for a wide range of complaints such as epileptic fits, melancholia, heart problems and nervous illnesses of all sorts.

> The rind of the bitter orange is much esteemed to recreate the spirits ... strengthen stomach and brain and resist malignancy of humours.[56]

The essential oil has been found to have a sedative effect on the nervous system. As a nerve tonic it helps to relax, calm and regenerate. It is also beneficial for those suffering from lack of energy or depression. The fragrance is fresh, warm and tangy. It adds roundness to most blends and makes a joyful, warming room fragrance for use in the home.

Like mandarin, the familiar sweet scent of orange is a favourite with children. It conveys a sense of lightheartedness and good cheer, and orange-peel pomanders have traditionally been used at Christmas and other festive occasions.

N.B. Mandarin oil (*C. reticulata*) shares many of the same properties as orange.

SCENT:
Citrus, fresh, fruity, radiant, sensual, sweet, tangy, warm. It blends well with lavender, lemon, neroli, petitgrain and spicy oils.

KEY QUALITIES:
Comforting, refreshing, sedative, soothing, tonic (nervous), uplifting, warming.

CONTRA-INDICATIONS:
The distilled (but not the expressed) oil is phototoxic. Can cause skin irritation in concentration; may cause an allergic reaction in some individuals.

Applications & Methods of Use:

- Add up to 5 drops to an evening bath to help soothe nervous anxiety, PMT, insomnia, emotional exhaustion and other stress-related problems. Use up to 3 drops for children's baths.
- For a soothing massage, orange blends well with neroli and petitgrain – add approx. 2 drops of each to 1 Tbs sweet almond oil.
- Dried orange peel, or the oil, is a traditional pot pourri ingredient. To make a scented pomander, stick an orange with cloves to sweeten the wardrobe and linen and keep moths away.

PATCHOULI *Pogostemon cablin*

Used to scent shawls, linen and clothes in India, patchouli is also dried in sachets to protect cloth and to scent the home. As a fumigant, it prevents the spread of disease and infection, and in Japan, China and Malaysia it is used in the treatment of various ailments, including headaches and nausea. In the East it was used as a remedy against insects and snake-bite, and is still employed as an insecticide and antiseptic.

Patchouli was first known in Britain in the 1820s when imported Indian shawls impregnated with patchouli oil became fashionable. Home imitations were unsaleable unless they too were scented with patchouli. It again attained popularity in the West during the 1960s, when it became associated with the hippy travellers to the East, who took to wearing the oil as a perfume. Most people tend to have a very strong reaction to the smell – they either love it or hate it. This may be due to individual temperament as well as its strong associations with the Orient.

Patchouli stimulates the nervous system in small doses, but is sedative in larger amounts. It has a marked aphrodisiac effect which, like ginseng, may be due to its effect on the endocrine glands. It is useful for depression, frigidity, anxiety and all stress-related conditions. Its rich, warm, musky fragrance has an appeasing, calming yet uplifting effect on the mind. It has an earthy, grounding quality, which according to Patricia

Scent:
Diffusive, earthy, medicinal, musky, oriental, powerful – improves with age, spicy, warm, woody.
It blends well with bergamot, cedarwood, lavender, myrrh, neroli, sandalwood, vetiver and other orientals.

Key Qualities:
Antiseptic, aphrodisiac, appeasing, calming, nerve tonic, sedative in large doses, stimulant in small amounts, uplifting.

Contra-indications:
Its over-use can cause loss of appetite, insomnia and nervous attacks.

Davis, 'is especially valuable for "dreamers" and people who tend to neglect or feel detached from their physical bodies'.[57]

In aromatherapy it is also used as a skin-care remedy, due to its excellent antiseptic and fungicidal properties.

Applications & Methods of Use:

- Add 5–10 drops to an evening bath to soothe anxiety, refresh the spirit and create a sensual mood.
- Used in a vaporizer, the oil makes a warm, exotic and relaxing room fragrance. It also prevents the spread of infection and repels insects.
- Mix 6 drops of patchouli with 1 Tbs sweet almond oil as a sensual massage oil. Massage clockwise slowly into the solar plexus to relieve stress.
- Wear neat as a long-lasting perfume for a rich, oriental appeal. Patchouli blends well with other oriental scents, especially sandalwood. (A few drops of oil added to the final hair rinse gives it an intriguing aroma and also helps combat dandruff.)
- The oil can be used for pot pourris and in sachets for scenting clothes and linen – it deters moths and is a good fixative. (The dried leaves or powder can also be bought.)

PEPPERMINT

– see Mint

PEPPER, BLACK 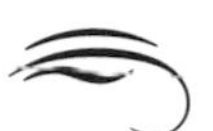 *Piper nigrum*

Black pepper is a very ancient spice, prized in the Far East for over 4,000 years and in Europe since the fifth century AD. It is mentioned in old Sanskrit and Chinese texts from the tenth century BC and still features highly in Indian Ayurvedic medicine. It was used by the Egyptians for cooking and therapeutic purposes. The presence of black pepper corns in the nostrils and abdomen of the mummy of Rameses II also indicates that it was used in the embalming process.

Of all the spices, pepper is probably the oldest trade item to travel the spice route from the Orient. Like the Egyptians, the Greeks and Romans used pepper both as a medicine and as a condiment. The Romans especially considered it an extremely valuable commodity and supplies of it were kept in huge storehouses, known as *borrea piperataria*, in Rome. Theophrastus and Dioscorides both extolled its virtues – Pliny recorded that pepper was more expensive to buy than gold! Tributes or taxes would commonly be paid in pepper corns in the ancient world, and the fortunes of Venice and Genoa were made through the wealth of the trade in pepper alone.

In medieval England, pepper was included in charms and amulets as a protection, probably because it was used as an antidote to poison, and to prevent the spread of infection. According to Culpeper, it is under Mars, having a hot, dry, fiery nature. It is a powerful tonic, having a strengthening effect on the entire system, especially the circulation, digestion, muscles and nerves. Joseph Miller says:

> It strengthens the nerves and head, and helps the sight; outwardly it is good for the tooth-ache, and for cold afflictions of the nerves, and pains in the limbs.[58]

SCENT:
Active, fresh, masculine, oriental, sensual, spicy, sporty, terpenic, warm, woody.
It blends well with frankincense, lavender, marjoram, rosemary, sandalwood, spices and florals.

KEY QUALITIES:
Analgesic, antiseptic, aphrodisiac, comforting, restoriative, stimulant (mental), strengthening, tonic (nerve).

CONTRA-INDICATIONS:
The oil is a skin irritant and toxic in concentration – use in low dilutions only (not more than ½ per cent in a blend).

Pepper is an excellent remedy for fatigue, whether mental or physical, and has the ability to increase endurance levels. Roman soldiers stationed in Britain are known to each have carried a small bag of pepper on their long marches. It is said that Buddhist monks in the Himalayas also take peppercorns with them on a tiring journey, to give them strength and alleviate hunger. In rural areas of India, powdered black pepper is given as an inhalation in cases of fainting and hysteria.

In aromatherapy, the oil is used to treat headache, neuralgia, nervous exhaustion and muscle fatigue. It is also an excellent antiseptic, bactericidal and analgesic oil. The warm, penetrating odour has an intellectually stimulating effect that increases alertness and concentration. Pepper has a warming, comforting quality which makes it useful for extreme cold, either of a physical or emotional nature. It has also been described as an aphrodisiac, probably due to its powerful stimulating effect.

> The chemical oil is an incomparable remedy, internally or externally, in weakness of the parts of generation of men or women … a few drops of the oil in any proper liniment (not stronger than ½% dilution!) rubbed upon the perineum 3 or 4 times will restore a lost erection.[59]

APPLICATION & METHODS OF USE:

- For headache and dullness caused by a hangover or overwork, put 3 drops each of pepper and juniper in a hot bath and inhale the vapours. Never use more than 3 drops of pepper in the bath.
- An effective treatment for neuralgia and general nervous or mental weakness is to blend 3 drops each of pepper, rosemary and

marjoram with 3 tsps of sweet almond oil and use as a massage oil. Massage slowly. This is especially good for athletes to soothe aches and pains and tone the muscles.

- In cooking, pepper mixed with hyssop, ginger and thyme is said to improve the sexual appetite. The French consider that adding plenty of freshly grated pepper to food as a condiment has a similar effect!
- A hint of pepper added to home perfumes, especially floral types, adds a zest to the blend – but take care not to use too much.
- As a vaporized oil, pepper is stimulating, reviving, warm and aids alertness, so use in combination with other oils such as basil or rosemary to increase concentration and fighting fatigue.

PINE, SCOTCH  *Pinus sylvestris*

The needles, bark, sawdust, resin, buds, cones and kernels of pine have all been utilized for their therapeutic properties throughout the ages, and many varieties of pine and fir are used to produce essential oils. The ancient Egyptians ate the pine kernels, which were considered restorative, in bread. The kernels were also used by the Romans, probably for food as well as a medicine. In his *Natural History*, Pliny described the therapeutic benefits of pine in great detail, especially with regard its effect on the respiratory tract. The dried needles were used to stuff mattresses by the American Indians, while the young tops were made into a type of beer which prevented scurvy. The twigs were mixed with equal parts of cedar and juniper and used as a purification incense, while the cones were considered fertility charms. Pine needle mattresses are still used as a folk remedy in the Swiss Alps for rheumatism. In Europe, young macerated shoots were added to the bath for nervous exhaustion and the sawdust was applied as a poultice along the spine for general debility. According to Culpeper, pine is governed by Jupiter and 'is of a mollifying, healing and cleansing nature'.[60]

Pine and fir are still very popular in bath preparations, due to their fresh scent and anti-rheumatic and anti-neuralgic properties. The fragrance alone stimulates the adrenal cortex and is an excellent pulmonary antiseptic. It also repels lice and fleas.

Pine needle oil, extracted from the needles of the Scotch pine, has a stimulating and invigorating effect on the circulation, yet its pleasing balsamic fragrance is soothing to the mind and good for anxiety and nervous tension. In addition, the scent of pine, for many people, conjures up the image of a natural wilderness of endless forests, thus evoking an open, expansive type of feeling. This makes it a useful oil for stress-related complaints, especially when accompanied by exhaustion and constant tiredness and when recovering from debilitating illness.

N.B. There are numerous different types of pine, fir and spruce used to produce essential oils, such as the longleaf pine (*Pinus palustris*), Siberian fir (*Abies sibirica*) or the Norway spruce (*Picea abies*), which share common properties. The Scotch pine needle oil, however, is one of the safest for therapeutic purposes. Some types of pine, such as dwarf pine (*Pinus pumilol*), are not recommended for therapeutic use at all.

SCENT:
Balsamic, fresh, masculine, penetrating, sporty, strong, turpenic, woody.
It blends well with juniper, lavender, lemon, marjoram, myrtle, rosemary and other woody oils.

KEY QUALITIES:
Cleansing, refreshing, restorative, reviving, soothing (mental), stimulant (nerve), strengthening.

CONTRA-INDICATIONS:
Skin irritant in concentration – use in dilution only.

APPLICATIONS & METHODS OF USE:

- An invigorating morning bath oil, having a tonic, reviving effect. Add up to 5 drops to the bath.
- An excellent bath oil to use after sport to soothe the muscles and help unwind after vigorous exercise, especially in combination with marjoram and juniper. Add 3 drops of each oil to the bath and relax.
- As an incense, it has a purifying, clean odour which combines well with other woods or resins, such as cedar, juniper or cypress. As a meditation aid, it helps clear the head and keep the mind alert.

- Pine oil makes a refreshing room fragrance, either used in a burner or added to pot pourris. It also kills germs, fights respiratory infection and repels insects – useful in the kitchen, bathroom or bedroom.
- Apart from birch, pine is the most traditional sauna scent, reminiscent of the vast evergreen forests of Scandinavia. Pine also aids the elimination of toxins through the skin – add a few drops to water thrown on the coals of the stove.
- For massage, pine is best used in combination with other tonic oils for nervous debility, lack of energy or emotional exhaustion, e.g. 2 drops each of pine, rosemary and juniper in 1 Tbs. sweet almond oil.

ROSE *Rosa centifolia* and *Rosa damascena*

There are three main types of traditional rose – the apothecary rose (*R. gallica*), which originated in Caucasus and was once used extensively in medicine; the cabbage rose (or Provence rose) which originated in Persia and is now grown extensively in Morocco; and the damask rose, a native of Syria, which has been cultivated in Bulgaria for about 300 years. They share many common qualities, although the French/Moroccan rose has a more narcotic effect than the Bulgarian type and has been shown to be a more potent aphrodisiac! The essence of the oriental or tea rose (*R. indica*) is also used in the East as a perfume and remedy.

The rose has been prized by all cultures alike. In Western myth, the rose is said to have sprung from the blood of Adonis, the Turks believe it came from the blood of Venus, while the Mohammedans say that it originated from the sweat of Mohammed. It has been associated with beauty and love for thousands of years, due to the perfection of its form and the allure of its scent. The white rose symbolizes purity and the red rose passion – a tradition still very much alive today. The rose has been called 'The Queen of Flowers'.

It is thought that the cultivation of the rose was spread throughout the world by the Arab nomads. It is probable that it was introduced into

Egypt in the reign of Rameses the Great. Remains of roses have been found in Egyptian tombs. A red rose is painted on the 4,000-year-old palace at Knossos in Crete.

The Romans scattered rose petals during banquets and threw them in the paths of their victors, they celebrated weddings and mourned funerals with wreaths of roses, and even wore rose garlands at their feasts to prevent drunkenness. They put petals in their baths and in their wine, as a perfume and as a remedy for hangover! Virgil records that Aphrodite requested that Hector's body be embalmed with rose essence. In AD 220 Athenaeus mentions that rose petals were strewn eight inches deep upon the ground when Cleopatra first met Mark Antony. Nero also used vast quantities of dried rose petals in his chambers.

To the early Christian mystics, the rose was associated with the Virgin Mary and 'divine love'. It was also the adopted symbol of the mystical Rosicrucian order. The Islamic esoteric Sufi tradition also venerated the rose as a symbol of transcendent desire. In the Hindu tradition, rose oil is frequently blended with sandalwood to form an oil called *aytar* for ritual use.

In Europe, during the Middle Ages, the rose was grown in monastery gardens and used as a strewing herb – it was one of the sixteenth-century English agriculturist Tusser's original strewing herbs – a perfume and as a herbal 'simple' (home remedy) especially for women's ailments:

> Red roses strengthen the heart … and procure rest and sleep … Red rose water is cooling, cordial, refreshing, quickening the weak and faint spirits, used either in meats or broths or to wash the temples, to smell at the nose, or to smell the sweep vapours out of a perfume pot, or cast into a hot fire-shovel.[61]

SCENT:
Floral, rich, rosy, sweet, tenacious, tender, warm. It blends well with bergamot, chamomile, clary sage, geranium, jasmine, lavender, neroli, patchouli and sandalwood.

KEY QUALITIES:
Anti-depressant, aphrodisiac, appeasing, comforting, regulating, sedative (nerve), soothing, tonic (heart), uplifting.

CONTRA-INDICATIONS:
Best avoided during the first four months of pregnancy.

An ointment of roses was used to soothe headaches, a syrup to 'comfort the heart', and rose leaves mixed with mint were applied externally as a poultice to 'quiet the over-heated spirits'. The fragrance of rose goes directly to the brain – important in the fighting of headaches and migraine. It is also good for hangovers!

In aromatherapy, rose essence is used as good general tonic and fortifier, particularly for the heart. It has a soothing action on the nerves, yet is a gentle aphrodisiac, especially for women. According to Patricia Davis, it is especially valuable for women who lack confidence or who are 'not secure' in their own sexuality. Scott Cunningham advocates the use of rose oil in visualization to manifest loving relationships. It has a comforting, sweet and uplifting fragrance, and a cephalic effect on the mind:

> Oleum rosarum (the oil of roses) is a good perfume; a drop or two cheers the heart, brain, animal and vitall spirits.[62]

Psychologically, the scent of rose can have a powerful effect, increasing concentration. It is also a mild sedative and anti-depressant, excellent for emotional shock, bereavement, grief and the treatment of melancholy – 'the rose distils a healing balm, the beating pulse of pain to calm'. Madame Maury recommends it as a means of regulating the appetite and overcoming obesity. She also has this to say about the essence of rose:

> But the rose procures us one thing above all: a feeling of well being, even of happiness, and the individual under its influence will develop an amiable tolerance.[63]

Applications & Methods of Use:

- Wear as a perfume to create a sensual mood. The effect of the fragrance also soothes nervous tension and helps overcome emotional stress, especially 'problems of the heart' such as loss, frigidity, grief, jealousy, shock, etc.
- For depression, post-natal depression, mood swings, PMT and menopausal problems, make a massage oil using 1 drop of rose in 1 tsp almond oil and rub gently into the solar plexus, back of the neck and temples.

- Add a few drops of oil to an evening bath to soothe the spirits and induce restful sleep. A rose-scented morning bath helps ease headaches and lift hangovers. A very 'safe' oil, which can also be used for children.
- The vaporized oil creates a romantic, warm atmosphere. Set the scene for seduction … or simply relax after a stressful day. Rose is also a good antiseptic and anti-infectious agent.
- Rose water applied to the temples and face is not only excellent for the complexion, but also reviving to the spirits and good for nervous headaches, dizziness or faintness.
- Rose petals or oil are traditionally used in pot pourris and also used for scenting sheets, linen, clothes, etc.

ROSEMARY *Rosmarinus officinalis*

An ancient medicinal herb, highly esteemed by East and West alike. The early Egyptians were familiar with it and used it as a ritual cleansing incense. Traces have been found in First Dynasty tombs. To the Greeks and Romans it was a sacred plant, symbolizing both love and death. They used it at all types of religious ceremonies – weddings, feasts and funerals. Sprigs are still carried traditionally at funerals and also at weddings or any occasions where solemn vows or pledges are made. In the West, rosemary has been associated for centuries with faithfulness, friendship and constancy, as in Ophelia's much quoted line from *Hamlet*:

> There's rosemary, that's for remembrance.[64]

It is also said that Greek students twined rosemary in their hair while studying for examinations! Rosemary was also known to the early Arabian physicians, and in Asia it was commonly grown on the graves of ancestors to invoke their help and guidance for the living. Conversely, in the West, a sprig of rosemary was carried to ward off evil spirits – a tradition still continued by the gypsies, who hang it up at their door as a protection.

First mentioned in an Anglo-Saxon herbal of the eleventh century, rosemary was one of the most popular aromatics used throughout Europe in the kitchen, still room, bedroom and garden. The dried herb was commonly burned as a purifying incense and a protection against contagious disease, including the plague. In France it was used as a fumigant in hospitals and sick rooms to disinfect the air. An old French name for it is *incensier*, for it was also burned in French churches and cathedrals.

It was sold in the apothecary's shop as a cure for hangovers and to restore youthfulness:

> See thee much Rosemary, and bathe therein to make thee lusty, lively, joyfull, likeing and youngly.[65]

The Elizabethans used it as a strewing herb and in place of smelling salts to revive a weak spirit. It is also one of the principal ingredients of 'Queen of Hungary water' (1370), renowned for its rejuvenating qualities. A garland of rosemary hung around the neck was recommended against 'the stuffing of the head and a cold braine', and a bundle of dried leaves bound in a cloth around the right arm were worn to make the mind 'light and merrie'. The dried leaves were placed under the pillow to protect from nightmares (especially for children), and were put in drawers and cupboards to keep moths at bay. Culpeper considered rosemary a herb of the sun, having many virtues:

> The decoction of rosemary in wine helps the cold distillations of rheums into the eyes, and other cold diseases of the head and brain, as the giddiness and swimmings therein, drowsiness or dulness, the dumb palsy [paralysis], or loss of speech, the lethargy, the falling sickness [epilepsy], to be drunk and the temples bathed there-with ... It helps weak memory and quickens the senses. The chymical [essential] oil drawn from the leaves and flowers, is a sovereign help for all the diseases aforesaid, to touch the temples and nostrils with two or three drops for all the diseases of the head and brain spoken of before ... yet it must be done with discretion, for it is very quick and piercing, and therefore but a little must be taken at a time.[66]

Rosemary water applied to the temples was used to relieve nervous headache. In medical herbalism, rosemary is still recommended for depression and nervous debility.

In aromatherapy, the oil is used as a tonic for the nerves, heart and circulation. It is a very effective nerve stimulant, good for all types of nervous debility, including loss of memory, lethargy and general dullness. It seems to improve the alertness and strength of all the senses – and has a marked cephalic effect! It has a refreshing, invigorating scent which has a reviving, uplifting effect on the spirit and helps dispel confusion and give the mind clarity. It has a pronounced action on the brain and is a classic remedy for fainting, headache, migraine and dizziness.

Rudolf Steiner thought that rosemary fortified the vital centre of an individual and increased the activity of the whole metabolism. Valnet recommends the essence of rosemary for cardiac complaints of nervous origin, such as palpitations, and for aphrodisiac and fortifying baths.

APPLICATIONS & METHODS OF USE:

- For a restorative, fortifying morning bath, good for hangovers, add 8–10 drops to the water. Also beneficial for children – use 5 drops only.
- A tonic massage oil can be made by mixing 6 drops of rosemary oil with 1 Tbs of almond oil and massaging clockwise into the solar plexus, chest or temples – good for general exhaustion, palpitations, headaches and other symptoms of stress.
- To rekindle lost energy, put one tsp of the dried herb in a pint (600 ml) of boiling water, let steep and sip slowly with honey.
- Inhale the vapour by putting a few drops in an oil burner or on a hanky for headaches, migraine, dizziness, mental and physical tiredness. This is also good for respiratory complaints of nervous origin, such as asthma.
- Burn the oil in a vaporizer or as an

SCENT:
Camphoraceous, fresh, penetrating, strong, woody-balsamic.
It blends well with elemi, juniper, lavender, myrtle, pine, thyme and spicy oils.

KEY QUALITIES:
Analgesic, protective, purifying, refreshing, restorative, reviving, stimulant (nerve and mental), strengthening, tonic (nerve).

CONTRA-INDICATIONS:
Not to be used during pregnancy or by epileptics.

incense for meditation, as it promotes clarity of mind. It also purifies the environment on a physical and psychic level.

- Put a few drops of oil or a sprig of rosemary in drawers or linen closets to keep away moths.

SAGE, CLARY *Salvia sclarea*

The generic name *Salvia* is derived from the Latin *salvaro* or *salveo*, meaning 'to save', due to the plant's ancient 'cure-all' reputation. The medicinal use of sage dates back to well before the birth of Christ: the early Egyptians recommended it for infertility and it was a popular herb with the Greeks and Romans, who believed that it ensured long life – it was called *herba sacra*, or 'sacred herb', by the Romans. The Greeks dedicated it to Zeus and the Romans to Jupiter, and it was the symbol of domestic virtue. An infusion of sage was taken as a tonic, a stimulant and blood purifier. Sage was also thought to banish all grief from the mind and body, and it was one of the most popular drinks in Britain before Indian and China teas were imported. Ironically, the Chinese preferred sage tea, for they claimed it conferred longevity.

In 1597 Gerard wrote:

> It is singularly good for the head and brain, it quicknethe the senses and memory, strengtheneth the sinews, restoreth health to those that have the palsy (paralysis), and taketh away shaky tremblings of the members.[67]

Clary sage was also formerly regarded as a very important medicinal herb, commonly known as 'clear eye' and employed for dimness of sight. It was already cultivated extensively in England by the sixteenth century, mainly for use in brewing ales. The botanist Lobel records that it made the beer more heady, causing those who drank it to become 'either dead drunk, or foolish drunk, or madde drunk'. Clary was also used to adulterate German wines, making them more intoxicating! It was also suggested that the seeds 'being beaten to powder and drank with wine, [are] an admirable help to provoke lust … '

The essential oil of clary sage shares many of the same properties of the

SCENT:
Amber, mellow, musky, reminiscent of ambergris, sweet.
Blends well with bergamot, cypress, geranium, jasmine, lavender, orange and sandalwood.

KEY QUALITIES:
Aphrodisiac, balancing, euphoric, inspiring, intoxicating, rejuvenating, relaxing, revitalizing, sedative (nerve).

CONTRA-INDICATIONS:
Do not use clary oil in combination with alcohol (i.e. do not drink for a few hours either before or after using clary); avoid during pregnancy.

common sage oil, but it is much safer. The oil from the common sage contains large amounts of thujone, which can provoke epileptic fits and in large quantities is toxic to the central nervous system. Clary sage oil contains a far lower proportion of thujone and is therefore used in aromatherapy in preference to the other types of sage.

Like common sage, clary contains an oestrogenic principle and helps restore nervous equilibrium. This makes it valuable for emotional or hormonal imbalance caused by PMT, the menopause or mid-life crisis. It is also a powerful nerve tonic, valuable for all types of nervous debility and states of exhaustion.

On a psychological level, the use of clary seems to encourage vivid dreams and enhance creative work due to its narcotic effect. It regenerates energy, and inspires both mind and spirit. Like bay, it can induce a kind of euphoria or a feeling of elation, although in some cases it simply causes drowsiness. It has a soothing, nutty, herbaceous odour which has a relaxing yet uplifting effect on the mind. The scent of clary sage can also bring about a sense of calmness or confidence in stressful situations, such as before an exam or interview. Maggie Tisserand highly recommends the oil in baths for over-excited, fretful or anxious children. As an aphrodisiac, it is useful for frigidity by helping to overcome apprehension or anxiety. Indeed, it is one of the most useful oils for all types of stressful conditions, deeply relaxing in effect.

APPLICATIONS & METHODS OF USE:

- For an excellent relaxing evening bath, add 5–10 drops to the water. Beneficial for all types of stress-related complaints, including insomnia, nervous exhaustion, headaches, migraine, fear, mental strain, irritability and anxiety. For children use up to 5 drops only.
- A tonic tea made from common sage is good for general debility, listlessness and promoting well-being: add a dessertspoonful of dried leaves to a pint (600 ml) of boiling water, let steep, then add honey to taste.
- Mix 6 drops of clary with 1 Tbs of sweet almond oil and massage clockwise into the solar plexus and spine to help menopausal problems, moods swings, PMT and other emotional or nervous afflictions, including depression and post-natal depression.
- Put a few drops of clary sage on the pillow or in a burner to encourage vivid dreams.
- The vaporized oil has an uplifting, relaxing effect – excellent during labour and for soothing the nerves.
- A sprig of sage in the wardrobe will keep away moths – the vaporized oil is also good for preventing the spread of airborne germs.

N.B. Spanish sage oil (*S. lavendulaefolia*) also makes a good alternative to common sage oil. Common sage is best avoided for therapeutic use.

SANDALWOOD 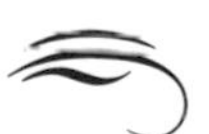 *Santalum album*

> In the Hindu marriage ceremony, the sacred fire is kept constantly burning … with sandalwood, perfumed oils, and incense which give off fragrant fumes.[68]

Used in India for thousands of years, sandalwood is mentioned in the oldest Vedic works from the fifth century BC. The wood was used to build temples, for it is immune to attack from white ants, and to carve idols and objects of art. The oil was employed in cosmetics and perfumes, and used to embalm the princes of Ceylon in the ninth century. Powdered sandalwood is much used as an incense in India and employed extensively in religious ceremonies such as the rituals of Vishnu. It is often traditionally combined with rose otto (in a blend called *aytar*). This is used, for example, on the last day of the Hindu year (12 April) to purify body and soul, and wash away sins of the past year. Sandalwood oil is still used widely in Indian Ayurvedic system of medicine, often in association with cardamom. Sandalwood was imported from India by the ancient Egyptians, who used it for embalming and as an incense, as well as for medical and cosmetic purposes.

In Tantric philosophy, sandalwood is recommended for men only, and is used to awaken the *kundalini* energy and transform it into enlightened mind. Indian yogis describe sandalwood as the fragrance of the 'subtle body'. The Japanese burn sandalwood and eagle wood on their Buddhist shrines, and during Shinto ceremonies; it also features in ancient Chinese texts. In Tibetan medicine, it is used in combination with other aromatics as a massage oil or incense for insomnia, anxiety and various psychological symptoms.

In Moslem countries, sandalwood and other ingredients are placed in a censer at the foot of the dead to carry their soul to heavenward. The rich use sandalwood to anoint their dead and burn it on their pyres – the poor must use juniper.

In aromatherapy, sandalwood is a valuable oil. It is a good antiseptic, having a gentle sedative, tonic effect on the nerves. It has an elevating, grounding and opening effect on the psyche, so is beneficial for depression, anxiety and stress-related problems. Avicenna wrote that the scent of sandalwood 'heals passions of the heart and doth exhilarate'. Its soft, balsamic, slightly spicy scent is relaxing, uplifting and even euphoric, which helps to account for why it is renowned as an aphrodisiac in the East. More recently, scientists have discovered that it contains a constituent similar to androsterone, the male underarm secretion which acts as a sexual signal.

East Indian sandalwood is also one of the most important ingredients of oriental perfumes and is an excellent fixative.

N.B. Poorer quality oils are produced from the Australian sandalwood (*S. spicatum*) used to make joss sticks in China and cheap perfumes, and amyris (*Amyris balsamifera*), used in soaps.

> SCENT:
> *Amber, balsamic, dry woody, masculine, musky, oriental, sensual, tenacious, warm. It blends well with benzoin, frankincense, jasmine, lemon, rose and ylang ylang.*
>
> KEY QUALITIES:
> *Aphrodisiac, elevating, grounding, opening, purifying, relaxing, sedative (nerve), soothing, uplifting, warming.*

APPLICATIONS & METHODS OF USE:

- Add 5–10 drops to the bath for insomnia, anxiety, depression, nervous tension, frigidity and other stress-related conditions.
- Use as an incense for yoga, meditation, etc. – it has a purifying and elevating effect.
- The vaporized oil makes a very pleasing room fragrance which is soothing to the nerves. Use in the bedroom to create an exotic, sensual atmosphere.
- For a relaxing, sensual massage, mix 2 drops each of sandalwood, jasmine and ylang ylang with 1 Tbs almond oil.
- Sandalwood oil makes a delicious perfume and a natural aphrodisiac, especially if worn by men.
- Its long-lasting fragrance is a pleasant addition to pot pourris. Sheets scented with sandalwood smell wonderful and help induce restful sleep.

SPIKENARD

see Valerian

TEA TREE

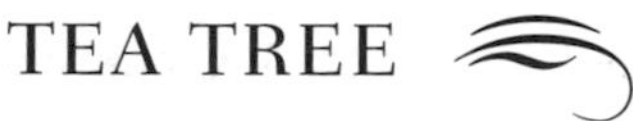

see Eucalyptus

THYME, COMMON  *Thymus vulgaris*

Thyme was one of the first medicinal plants employed throughout the Mediterranean region. It was used by the ancient Egyptians in the embalming process and by the Sumerians as long ago as 3500 BC. The ancient Greeks used thyme to fumigate against infectious illness; the name derives from the Greek *thymos*, meaning 'to perfume'. It was offered to Venus and other divinities as an incense. The Romans bathed in thyme to give them vigour and courage, an idea which continued to the time of the Crusades, when ladies would embroider their knights' scarves with sprigs of thyme before going into battle. It was also considered a prime remedy for melancholy. Pliny recommended it for epilepsy; he also said that a mattress or pillow stuffed with dried thyme would make a patient relaxed and calm.

Common thyme was cultivated in England by the middle of the sixteenth century for medicinal and culinary use, although the wild species, known as the 'Mother of Thyme' (*T. serpyllum*) was known much earlier. It was used with a sprig of parsley and a few bay leaves to scent and soften bath water. Thyme was also grown as a popular 'bee plant' in gardens and it was a favourite strewing herb. The oil was distilled in many country still rooms, mainly due to its excellent antiseptic properties. As a fumigant, it was considered to be a herb of purification and cleansing, and was also thought to 'enliven the spirits' by its fragrance. Culpeper has this to say about the wild thyme:

> The whole plant is very fragrant and yields an essential oil that is very heating. An infusion of the leaves removes headache, occasioned by inebriation. It is under Venus, and is excellent for nervous disorders. A strong infusion, drank as tea, is pleasant, and a very effectual remedy for headache, giddiness and other disorders of that kind: and a certain remedy for that troublesome complaint, the nightmare.[69]

During the eighteenth century, thyme was included in many preparations for nervous disorders, including *baume tranquille*, used for hysteria and other psychological complaints. It was highly thought of as a 'brain fortifier' and a nerve tonic which helped to re-establish strength during convalescence. It was also thought to 'resist madness and all diseases of melancholy'.[70]

In aromatherapy, the essential oil is considered of prime use for warming, stimulating and fortifying the whole metabolism:

> It is helpful whenever inner warmth is poor or missing: excess of water, chilling tendencies, cold and weakness of the vital centre, especially when it is manifested at the level of lungs or stomach.[71]

Its penetrating herbaceous scent is anti-depressant and uplifting, having an energizing effect on the emotional, mental and physical levels.

N.B. There are many different varieties of thyme and essential oils produced from these different varieties of 'chemotypes' each contain a specific balance of constituents. There are the thymol-carvacrol types, which are hot and burning, the fragrant, citron-scented types and the milder 'linalol' types, such as the wild thyme or 'serpolet' oil. The latter two are less prone to be irritants.

The red thyme oil (thymol-carvacrol type) should be avoided.

SCENT:
Fresh, green, herbaceous, medicinal, penetrating, powerful, spicy, sporty, warm. It blends well with bergamot, lemon, marjoram, melissa, pine and rosemary.

KEY QUALITIES:
Antiseptic, purifying, refreshing, restorative, reviving, stimulating (mental), tonic (nerve), warming.

CONTRA-INDICATIONS:
The white thyme oil (which has been redistilled to remove irritant substances) should be used in moderation and in low dilution only. The 'citron' and 'linalol' types are safer for general use. All types should be avoided during pregnancy.

APPLICATIONS & METHODS OF USE:

- Add up to 5 drops to a morning bath for physical and mental debility, depression, lethargy and fatigue. Good for hangovers and headaches.
- The vaporized oil helps clear the head and is good for nervous headaches, anxiety, worry, mental chatter, etc. It has a purifying effect on both a physical and psychic level.

- Thyme is best used in combination with other tonic oils for massage to help to revive and strengthen both body and mind, e.g. 2 drops each of thyme, rosemary and black pepper in 1 Tbs almond oil.
- For a fortifying morning tea, especially good for convalescence, infuse a heaped Tbs fresh thyme leaves in 1 pint (600 ml) of boiling water, let steep and sweeten with honey.

VALERIAN *Valeriana officinalis*

Valerian was one of the ancient sacred herbs, a *benedicta* or blessed herb. The name derives from the Latin *valere*, 'to be well'. The root was prized in ancient Greek and Roman medicine as a powerful sedative and the Greeks are known to have hung bunches of the leaves on doors and windows as a protection. It is often described as having magical properties, and it was used both for and against witchcraft. It was thought to defend against thunder and lightening, and was used in love charms, as it was supposed to inspire love. It was later held sacred to the Virgin Mary and dedicated to St Bernard.

In the Middle Ages the powdered root was used not only as a medicine but also as a spice and a perfume. It was the custom to lay the roots among clothes, just as some of the Himalayan valerians are still used in the East to scent cloth and bath water. The Eastern varieties, known as *Nardus*, have a more pleasing scent than the Western varieties.

Spikenard, which is closely related to valerian, was one of the earliest aromatics used by the ancient Egyptians and Eastern civilizations. It is mentioned in the Song of Solomon and was the oil which Mary used to anoint Jesus before the Last Supper. 'Nard' was also used by European herbalists for 'it heals all old and cold diseases of the brain … tremblings, palsies, apoplexies, forgetfulness and sleepy diseases'.[72]

Valerian was used medicinally for all types of nervous affliction, including hysteria and epilepsy. Native American herbalists believe that if epileptic fits do not respond to this herb then they are incurable. It is still one of the most widely used nerve tonics in herbal medicine and often prescribed as a cure for insomnia, for it calms the mind without having a narcotic effect:

> Clinical studies of valerian show that it improves the quality of sleep as measured by subjective assessment by the patients themselves; this is confirmed to some extent by EEG. It reduced the time taken to fall asleep, particularly in older people and in habitually poor sleepers, and did not cause somnolence in the morning of affect dream recall.[73]

Its fragrance has a relaxing, slightly euphoric effect on the mind, although most people find its scent disagreeable – one of its old herbal names was 'phu'! The smell of this plant has a curious effect on some animals – cats become frisky and intoxicated. An oil prepared from valerian and aniseed is used by gypsies to quell unfriendly dogs. Horses are known to like its scent, as are rats and mice. It was once used as a bait in traps – and possibly by the Pied Piper of Hamelin!

N.B. Oil of spikenard (*Nardostachys jatamasi*) shares many of the properties of valerian.

SCENT:
Balsamic, earthy, green, musky, warm, woody. It blends well with cedarwood, lavender, marjoram, patchouli, petitgrain, pine and citrus oils.

KEY QUALITIES:
Calming, depressant of the central nervous system, grounding, mildly hypnotic, protective, regulator, sedative (mental and nervous), soothing.

CONTRA-INDICATIONS:
In large amounts, valerian can cause headaches, mental agitation and delusions. Use in moderation and do not use over long periods of time (more than a month without a break).

APPLICATIONS & METHODS OF USE:

- For an evening bath oil, add 5–10 drops to the water. Valerian is excellent for nervous exhaustion brought on by emotional excitement, anxiety, mental chatter, restlessness and stress-related disorders.
- The vaporized oil is good for nervous headaches, migraine and to generally soothe and calm the mind.

- A massage oil made by mixing 2 drops each of valerian, marjoram and lavender with 1 Tbs of base oil is excellent for nervous exhaustion, mental strain, tiredness and as a general tonic to the nervous system. It is especially effective when blended with other relaxants, such as chamomile or melissa. Beneficial for those of a nervous temperament.
- A tea or tisane can be made by soaking 1 tsp of powdered root in a cup of cold water for 12 hours, then straining it and drinking before retiring. It is an effective tranquillizer without any side-effects. It should not, however, be taken for longer than 3 or 4 weeks at a time – a fortnight's break is then recommended.

VETIVER 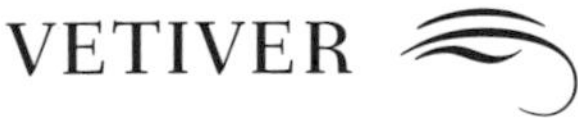 *Vetiveria zizanoides*

Vetiver or vetivert is a tropical or sub-tropical plant, closely related to other aromatic grasses such as lemongrass and citronella which share similar properties. Like its relatives, vetiver has been used throughout the ages as an insect repellent, but it is also renowned for its pleasing scent. In India, where it is known as *khus khus* or *khas khas*, small bundles or roots are put in wardrobes or woven into screens which are hung in windows and doorways to keep insects away while at the same time emitting a delightful fragrance. The essential oil is still used to scent cotton cloth, in the same way as patchouli, to protect it from moths. In Russia, little sachets impregnated with vetiver oil were attached to the lining of expensive fur coats for the same purpose.

But vetiver's main use has always been in perfumery, especially in the East. In India the powdered roots are used in oriental scents and incense; in the West it is used as a fragrance component in after-shaves and soaps, and as a fixative.

The warm earthy, slightly musky scent has a soothing and relaxing effect. In India and Sri Lanka the essence is known as 'oil of tranquillity', due to its calming and uplifting quality.

In aromatherapy, vetiver is recommended for all types of stress-related complaints, including insomnia, depression and anxiety. It has a grounding, earthy yet inspiring quality that makes it a good oil for use during meditation.

According to Patricia Davis, vetiver acts as a protection against over-sensitivity, or becoming a 'psychic sponge'. Mimosa oil is similar in this respect.

Some people consider the warm, earthy scent an aphrodisiac.

N.B. Lemongrass (*Cymbopogon citratus*) and citronella (*C. nardus*) share similar therapeutic properties, although are more strongly citrus scented.

SCENT:
Diffusive, dry woody, earthy, green, masculine, rich, smoky, sporty, sweet, warm. It blends well with clary sage, jasmine, lavender, patchouli, rose, sandalwood and ylang ylang.

KEY QUALITIES:
Calming, grounding, protective, sedative (nervous and mental), soothing, tonic (nervous), uplifting.

APPLICATIONS & METHODS OF USE:

- Add 5–10 drops to an evening bath to promote a peaceful state of mind.
- Best blended with other oriental relaxants for massage, e.g. 2 drops each of vetiver, sandalwood and ylang ylang in 1 Tbs sweet almond oil for a sensual, soothing experience.
- The vaporized oil makes a delightful calming room fragrance, excellent for the bedroom. It also can aid meditation, yoga, etc., and keeps insects at bay.
- The scent of the oil deters moths. For a pleasing alternative to moth balls, impregnate a piece of tissue or a hanky with the oil and place in drawers and/or in the linen closet.

YARROW *Achillea millefolium*

Yarrow is an age-old herbal remedy used for a wide variety of different complaints. It was considered sacred in the Germanic countries, especially as a herb for healing battle wounds. Its name derives from the Trojan war hero Achilles, who is said to have healed his Achilles tendon with this herb. According to Culpeper, it is a herb of Venus which 'induces sleep, eases the pain and lessens the bleeding'.[74]

In ancient China, it was considered a sacred plant and its stems were used to make the 50 sticks used for divination by the *I Ching*. In Chinese herbalism it was thought to represent a perfect balance between the yin and yang energies, hard and soft, the two polarities found in nature.

In the West it has also been associated with divination and magic. One of its old folk names is 'devil's plaything'. It was thought that an ounce of yarrow sewn in a bag and placed under the pillow would bring a vision of one's future husband or wife:

Thou pretty herb of Venus' tree
Thy true name it is yarrow;
Now who my bosom friend must be,
Pray tell thou me to-morrow.[75]

In medical herbalism it was once used for epilepsy, hysteria and trembling, as well as being an excellent fever and wound herb. It is still recognized as a valuable nerve tonic, for it strengthens and revitalizes the whole system. In the Orkneys the tea is considered a good remedy for melancholy. It is also taken in Germanic countries for depression and moodiness.

In aromatherapy, yarrow oil is used as a balancing remedy during the menopause.

SCENT:
Fresh, green, herbaceous, slightly camphoraceous, sweet, warm.
It blends well with chamomile, clary sage, hyssop, melissa, myrtle, valerian and vetiver.

KEY QUALITIES:
Balancing, grounding, mildly stimulating, opening, restorative, revitalizing, strengthening, tonic (nerve).

CONTRA-INDICATIONS:
Can cause skin irritation in concentration.

During hormonal changes it can help to keep psychological equilibrium intact and help reorganize the shifting energies.

It can also be used for nervous headaches, depression, exhaustion and stress-related problems.

Applications & Methods of Use:

- Add 5 drops to the bath for PMT, insomnia, nervous exhaustion and stress-related conditions.
- Best blended with other oils for massage, e.g. 2 drops each of clary sage, chamomile and yarrow for emotional imbalance or moodiness.
- For an uplifting, tonic tea, add 1 dessertspoonful of dried flowers to 1 pint (600 mls) of boiling water, let steep and add honey to taste.

YLANG YLANG 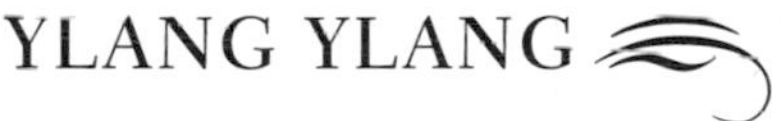 *Cananga odorata var. genuina*

This large exotic yellow flower emits a rich, sensual fragrance. The name means 'flower of flowers'. In 1866, Guibourt, in his *Histoire naturelle des drogues simples*, compared its scent to that of narcissus, being intoxicating and narcotic. In Indonesia, the flowers are spread on the beds of newly married couples on their wedding night. Ylang ylang has a long-standing reputation as a potent aphrodisiac, and its euphoric qualities can help overcome depression and apathy. PMT, menopausal problems and post-natal depression also respond well to this oil.

In aromatherapy, it is recommended for psychological or emotional difficulties, especially those connected with lack of confidence, frigidity in particular. Its powerful yet soothing scent helps overcome fear and encourages a relaxed attitude. This is also valuable in stressful situations in helping to deal with irritation, impatience or anxiety. R. W. Moncrieff observed:

> The writer working with odorous materials for more than twenty years, long ago noticed that … ylang ylang soothes and inhibits anger born of frustration.[76]

SCENT:
Balsamic, floral, heady, oriental, rich, sensual, slightly spicy, soft, sweet.
It blends well with bergamot, jasmine, rose, sandalwood, vetiver and other orientals.

KEY QUALITIES:
Aphrodisiac, appeasing, calming, euphoric, narcotic, regulating, sedative, soothing.

CONTRA-INDICATIONS:
Used in excess it can cause headaches or nausea.

On a physical level, it relaxes the central nervous system, having a sedating or even soporific effect. It is excellent for those suffering from high blood pressure, palpitations, insomnia and other symptoms of hypertension. It also has a regulating effect on the heart, on both a physical and emotional level.

N.B. Tuberose (*Polianthes tuberosa*) shares many of the same properties as ylang ylang, being heady, floral and narcotic. Not to be confused with cananga (*C. Odoratum var. macrophylla*), an inferior oil of a closely related species.

APPLICATION & METHODS OF USE:

- Add 5–10 drops to an evening bath to soothe irritation and renew energy; good for insomnia, nervous tension and all stress-related problems.
- For a sensual, relaxing massage, ylang ylang blends well with jasmine, rose or neroli. The aphrodisiac and uplifting effect is also beneficial for depression and frigidity and to help overcome other emotional constraints.
- The vaporized oil makes a soothing, heady room fragrance. A few drops on a hanky, inhaled periodically throughout the day, helps overcome nervousness.
- An intriguing perfume oil in its own right, rich and sensual. It has a lingering scent which clings to scarves, clothes and linen.

REFERENCES

1. Lovell, R., *A Compleat Herball*, 2nd edition, 1665, p.14.
2. Ibid.
3. Fischer-Rizzi, S., *The Complete Aromatherapy Handbook*, Sterling, 1990, p.60.
4. Lovell, op. cit. p.15.
5. Rapgay, L., *Tibetan Therapeutic Massage*, 1985, p.25.
6. Cited in Tisserand, R., *The Art of Aromatherapy*, C. W. Daniel, 1985, p.182.
7. Culpeper, N., *Culpeper's Complete Herbal*, W. Foulsham Co. Ltd., p.40.
8. Lovell, op. cit., p.35.
9. Joseph Miller, cited in Tisserand, R., *The Art of Aromatherapy*, C. W. Daniel, 1985, p.186.
10. Maury, M., *Marguerite Maury's Guide to Aromatherapy*, C. W. Daniel, 1989, p.96.
11. Davis, P., *Aromatherapy: An A–Z*, C. W. Daniel, 1985, p.204.
12. Fischer-Rizzi, op. cit., p.72.
13. Tisserand, R., op. cit., p.204.
14. Grieve, M., *A Modern Herbal*, Penguin Books, Middlesex, 1982, p.157.
15. Ibid., p.206.
16. Exodus 30: 22–5.
17. Parvati, J., *Hygieia, A Woman's Herbal*, Wildwood House, 1979, p.24.
18. Valnet, J., *The Practice of Aromatherapy*, C. W. Daniel, English translation, 1982, p.119.
19. Ryman, D., *The Aromatherapy Handbook, Century*, 1984, p.85.
20. Valnet, op. cit., p.119.
21. Ryman, op. cit., p.126
22. Lovell, R., *A Compleat Herball*, 2nd edition, 1665, p.119.
23. Davis, P., *Subtle Aromatherapy*, C. W. Daniel, 1991, p.203.
24. Lovell, op. cit., p.488.
25. Davis, op. cit., p.204.
26. le Strange, R., *A History of Herbal Plants*, Angus and Robertson, 1977, p.116.
27. Parvati, op. cit., p.123.
28. Exodus 30: 34–6.
29. Maury, M., *Marguerite Maury's Guide to Aromatherapy*, C. W. Daniel, 1989, p.104.
30. Lovell, op. cit., p.145.
31. Ryman, D., *Aromatherapy*, Piatkus, 1991, p.109.
32. de Baïracli, Levy, J., *The Illustrated Herbal Handbook*, Faber & Faber, 1974, p.92.
33. Psalms 51: 7.
34. Davis, op. cit., p.206.
35. Al-Kindi, *The Medical Formulary*, Wisconsin Press, 1966, p.190.
36. Culpeper, N., *Culpeper's Complete Herbal*, W. Foulsham Co. Ltd., p.202.

37. Lavabre, M., *Aromatherapy Workbook*, Healing Arts Press, 1990, p.69.
38. Davis, P., *Aromatherapy: An A–Z*, C. W. Daniel, 1988, p.191.
39. Fischer-Rizzi, S., *Complete Aromatherapy Handbook*, Sterling, 1990, p.151.
40. Ibid., p.120.
41. Culpeper, op. cit., p.216.
42. Ibid., p.227.
43. Ranson, F., *British Herbs*, Penguin, 1949, p.145.
44. Wren, R. C., *Potter's New Cyclopaedia of Botanical Drugs and Preparations*, C. W. Daniel, 1988, p.23.
45. Davis, P., *Subtle Aromatherapy*, C. W. Daniel, 1991, p.213.
46. Culpeper, op. cit., p.234.
47. Cited in Tisserand, R., *The Art of Aromatherapy*, C. W. Daniel, 1985, p.259.
48. Davis, op. cit., p.214.
49. Lovell, R., *A Compleat Herball*, 2nd edition, 1665, p.288.
50. Ryman, D., *Aromatherapy*, Piatkus, 1991, p.152.
51. Fischer-Rizzi, op. cit., p.139.
52. Sellar, W., *Aromatherapy Quarterly*, no.34, p.20.
53. Davis, P., *Aromatherapy: An A–Z*, C. W. Daniel, 1988, p.237.
54. Gordon, L., *A Country Herbal*, Webb & Bower, 1980, p.127.
55. le Strange, R., *A History of Herbal Plants*, Angus and Robertson, 1977, p.185.
56. Pomet, P., *A Compleat History of Druggs*, Lemery & Tournefort, 1712, p.152.
57. Davis, P., *Subtle Aromatherapy*, C. W. Daniel, 1991, p.217.
58. Cited in Tisserand, R., op. cit., p.193.
59. Pomet, op. cit., p.122.
60. Culpeper, N., *Culpeper's Complete Herbal*, W. Foulsham Co. Ltd., p.144.
61. Grieve, M., *A Modern Herbal*, Penguin Books, Middlesex, 1982, pp.300-1.
62. Lovell, op. cit., p.369.
63. Maury, M., *Marguerite Maury's Guide to Aromatherapy*, C. W. Daniel, 1989, p.87.
64. Hamlet, IV. v. 174.
65. Langham, W., *The Garden of Health*, 1579.
66. Culpeper, op. cit., p.303.
67. Cited in le Strange, A History of Herbal Plants, Angus and Robertson, 1977, p.218.
68. Thompson, C. J. S., *The Mystery and Lure of Perfume*, John Lane, 1927.
69. Culpeper, op. cit., p.372.
70. Lovell, R., *A Compleat Herball*, 2nd edition, 1665, p.436.
71. Lavabre, M., *Aromatherapy Workbook*, Healing Arts Press, 1990, p.79.
72. Lovell, op. cit., p.412.
73. Wren, R. C., *Potter's New Cyclopaedia of Botanical Drugs and Preparations*, C. W. Daniel, 1988, p.275.

74. Culpeper, op. cit., p.398.
75. Grieve, M., *A Modern Herbal*, Penguin Books, Middlesex, 1982, p.864.
76. Cited in Tisserand, R., The Art of Aromatherapy, C. W. Daniel, 1985, p.286.

Appendix I:

Useful Addresses

It is important to buy good quality essential oils if they are to be effective therapeutically. Synthetic perfume oils or dilute products do not have the same potency and cannot be substituted for 100 per cent pure and natural aromatic oils. There are now many brands of essential oils available but the quality control and ethical standard can vary.

Aqua Oleum have many years' experience in the field and provide a wide range of top quality essential oils at very competitive prices as well as a large selection of virgin-pressed carrier or base oils. They can be purchased from health and whole food stores throughout the United Kingdom, as well as from some chemists. Mail order items, individually formulated products, the 'Essential Oil Catalogue' and further information can be obtained from:

Aqua Oleum, Unit 3, Lower Wharf, Wallbridge, Stroud, Glos., GL5 3JA

Tel: 01453 753555

If you want to experience a professional aromatherapy treatment, it is vital that you choose a therapist who has undergone an accredited training. The International Federation of Aromatherapists ensures that its members have attained a recognized standard of practice and provides a list of qualified practitioners throughout the United Kingdom

For those wishing to further their interest in aromatherapy, the Federation also publishes a newsletter, holds open meetings and can recommend training programmes for individuals wishing to gain a professional qualification. They can be contacted at:

The International Federation of Aromatherapists, Department of Continuing Education, Royal Masonic Hospital, Ravenscourt Park, London W6 0TN

Tel: 0181–846 8066

Information regarding qualified medical herbalists and training programmes can be obtained from:

The School of Herbal Medicine/Phytotherapy, Bucksteep Manor, Bodle Street Green, Hailsham, Sussex, BN27 4RJ

Tel: 01323 833812/4

Appendix II:

Directions for Use and Safety Data

Tea or Tisane

The proper way to prepare a tisane or tea is to use the following method:

Place the required amount of the herb into a non-metal container – a teapot or thermos flask is the most effective.
Pour the required amount of boiling water over it.
Cover with a lid to prevent evaporation of important constituents – this is especially important with highly aromatic herbs.
Leave to steep or infuse for 5–10 minutes.

Proportions are:

30 g dried herb to ½ litre of boiling water; or
1 Tbs of fresh chopped herb to boiling water; or
½ Tbs dried herb to boiling water.
Seeds, roots or spices may need longer to infuse.

Baths

Bathing is a relaxing therapeutic experience in itself and can heighten the psychological effect of essential oils. It is the easiest and most popular way of using essential oils at home. Simply add between 5 and 10 drops of a chosen oil to the bath water when the tub is full and relax in the aromatic vapour. Different essential oils can be selected for their specific effect – rosemary is uplifting and stimulating; chamomile is soothing and relaxing. Essential oils can also be blended for bathing, but take care not to exceed 10 drops altogether.

Essential oils can also be mixed in a teaspoon of vegetable oil (such as sweet almond oil) before being added to the bath. This helps to moisturize the skin and ensure an even distribution of the essential oils, which is important in the case of babies and young children. Always check specific contra-indications before using a new oil in the bath, to avoid possible irritation.

Massage

Massage is one of the most potent stress-relieving treatments that we have at our disposal. This has been recognized by all cultures alike, and utilized as a means of keeping the mind as well as the body in a healthy condition. When aromatic oils are used as a part of this process, they are absorbed readily through the skin and dispersed into the air simultaneously – thus ensuring both a physiological and a psychological effect. Massage can also be a very sensual experience and massage between lovers can help bring a new depth to a relationship, as well as enhance sexual enjoyment.

Therapeutic massage is the main method used by professional aromatherapists, but it can equally well be practised at home, either on oneself, or by a friend or partner. If it is not possible to carry out a full body massage, then a foot massage using appropriate oils is an excellent alternative. When we massage the feet, we stimulate and affect all the rest of the body as well. This is because all the organs, glands and muscles in the human body have nerve endings located in the soles of the feet.

For the purpose of massage, essential oils are mixed with a carrier oil or vegetable oil such as sweet almond oil or grapeseed oil before being applied to the body. The dilution should be in the region of 1–3 per cent, depending upon the type of oils used and the specific purpose. Psychological complaints or those related to the emotions, such as depression, insomnia and stress, generally require a weaker concentration than disorders of a more physical nature.

An easy way of calculating how much essential oil to add to a base oil is to assess the amount of base oil in millilitres and then add about half the number of drops of essential oil. For example:

To a 50 ml bottle of base oil, add about 25 drops of essential oil – this gives a 2.5 per cent dilution. Add a few more drops for a physical remedy, a few less for the treatment of an emotional or psychological problem.

To 1 Tbs (approx. 15 ml) base oil, add 6–9 drops of essential oil.

To 1 tsp carrier oil (approx 5 ml), add 2–3 drops of essential oil.

Vaporized Oils

Vaporized oils are a convenient and smoke-free way of scenting a room for dispelling unwanted odours. Fragrances add atmosphere to the home and certain oils can be used to create a specific mood, such as for meditation, romance or for a festive occasion. Personal experimentation is all that is required!

There are many methods available for vaporizing essential oils, including using an oil burner or an electric diffuser, or by simply adding a few drops of oil to a bowl of hot water placed on a radiator. Avoid applying essential oil directly to a light bulb, as it can cause the bulb to explode. If you wish to keep insects at bay, then applying oil to hanging ribbons or to clothing can be very effective. Apply a few drops of an expectorant essential oil such as myrtle to the pillow, on pyjamas or a nightie, or on a hanky to help combat coughs and colds. These are all ways of ensuring that the vaporized oil will have an effect.

Perfumes and 'Individual Prescriptions'

Many essential oils are ideal as perfumes – either on their own or combined with others. Ylang ylang is renowned as a well-balanced fragrance in its own right; others, such as rose, jasmine, neroli and sandalwood are well-known traditional scents. Such oils can be dabbed on the wrist or behind the ears, either neat or diluted to 5 per cent in jojoba or a bland base oil. Before using an new oil as a perfume, always do a patch test first, i.e. apply a little to the wrists and wait for an hour to see whether any irritation occurs. If it does, rinse with warm water and reduce the concentration or avoid altogether in the future.

To make a personalized perfume or 'individual prescription', combine between 3 and 7 essential oils, according to need, in 50 per cent jojoba or 'light' coconut oil, and leave to mature for about a month. This will make a concentrated 'unguent'-style perfume which will not go rancid. For further details, see Chapter 6, The 'Individual Prescription'.

Aromatic oils can also be used to scent the hair, linen or clothes, paper, pot pourris or other items. Pure essential oils have a totally different quality from synthetic perfumes, since they are derived from natural sources. Artificially made perfumes do not have the subtle balance of constituents and the therapeutic qualities of real essential oils.

Safety Data

- Due to their high concentration, essential oils should not be taken internally. This corresponds with the International Federation of Aromatherapists code of practice.
- In general, essential oils should not be applied neat to the skin, due to their concentration. Some oils can cause irritation or a burning or tingling sensation when they are applied in an undiluted form. However, there are exceptions to this rule. Lavender can be applied directly to the skin, as can various perfume oils such as ylang ylang or jasmine (see contra-indications on each oil). Most oils should never be applied neat to the skin, unless specifically directed.
- Certain oils are contra-indicated during pregnancy, in cases of high blood pressure, epilepsy or depression. Always check specific contra-indications for each oil.
- Babies and children are more sensitive to the effects of essential oils than adults. Always apply essential oils in a higher dilution for children (half the amount of essential oil indicated for adults) and dissolve essential oils in milk or vegetable oils before adding to bath water. *All essential oils should be stored well out of the reach of children.*

Appendix III:

Astrological Correspondences

That remedies can either cure by sympathy or by antipathy is a principle recognized by contemporary medicine – the former in homoeopathy, the latter in allopathic medication. The same principle has also long been applied to the planetary correspondences ascribed to herbs and aromatics, and their use in herbal medicine and aromatherapy.

Sign	*Ruler*	*Element*	*Humour*	*Cross*
Aries	Mars+	fire	choleric	cardinal
Taurus	Venus-	earth	phlegmatic	fixed
Gemini	Mercury+	air	sanguine	mutable
Cancer	Moon	water	melancholic	cardinal
Leo	Sun	fire	choleric	fixed
Virgo	Mercury-	earth	phlegmatic	mutable
Libra	Venus+	air	sanguine	cardinal
Scorpio	Pluto/Mars-	water	melancholic	fixed
Sagittarius	Jupiter+	fire	choleric	mutable
Capricorn	Saturn-	earth	phlegmatic	cardinal
Aquarius	Uranus/Saturn+	air	sanguine	fixed
Pisces	Neptune/Jupiter-	water	melancholic	mutable

Correspondences between the astrological sign, the planet and the humour also provide information about the temperament of an individual, and what diseases or imbalances they are likely to suffer from. Lovell described the qualities of each planet in the following way, together with the parts they governed:

Sun: Hot and dry, a benevolent planet and friend to Jupiter and Venus. It governs the vital faculties, the heart and arteries.
Diseases include fainting, convulsions, heartburn and trembling.
Aromatics include angelica, balm, bay, chamomile, frankincense, lavender, marjoram, mastic, myrrh, orange, rose, rosemary, thyme and all the spices.

Moon: Cold and moist, a friend to Saturn, Jupiter, Venus and Mercury. It corresponds to the brain and is therefore sympathetic to the nervous system and vital spirits.
Diseases include sciatica, lethargic and phlegmatic complaints.
Aromatics include hyssop, lime, mastic and nutmeg.

Mercury: Mutable, a friend to Saturn, Jupiter, Venus and the Moon. It governs the imagination and intellect, the brain and vital spirits (together with the Sun and Moon), also the extremities, hands and feet.
Diseases include infatuation, stammering, epilepsy, vertigo, insanity, 'hurts of the intellect'.
Aromatics include aniseed, chamomile, cubeb, dill, fennel, juniper, lavender, savory, sweet marjoram, thyme, valerian.

Venus: Cold and moist, a friend to the Sun, Mars, Mercury and the Moon. It governs the genitals and 'feminine' characteristics.
Diseases include immoderate lust, infertility, frigidity, problems with menstruation and procreation, venereal disease.
Aromatics include clary sage, coriander, geranium, labdanum, mint, mugwort, musk, rose, sandalwood, thyme, violet and all perfumes.

Mars: Exceedingly hot and dry, a friend to Venus. It governs the nose and the sense of smell, which is 'hot and dry', also the bladder.
Diseases include epilepsy.
Aromatics include basil, garlic, hops, mustard and wormwood.

Jupiter: Hot and moist, a friend to all except Mars. It governs the liver, veins and lungs.
Diseases include respiratory disorders, choleric complaints.
Aromatics include basil, bay, mastic, mint, red rose, sage, spike, storax and violet.

Saturn: Cold and dry, a friend to Mars. It governs the head and the retentive faculties.
Diseases include melancholy, madness, grief, fear and loss of memory.
Aromatics include cumin, cypress, opium, parsley, pine and sage.

Planetary Correspondences*

Planet	Colour	Plant	Metal	Gem	Perfumes
Sun	Orange	Sunflower, heliotrope, chicory	Gold	Topaz, diamond	Aloe wood, saffron, cloves, cinnamon, myrrh
Moon	Violet	Hazel, almond, peony	Silver	Crystal, pearl, quartz	Camphor, jasmine, frankincense, white sandalwood
Mercury	Yellow	Vervain, palm, cinquefoil	Quicksilver	Agate, opal	Cinnamon, mace, cloves, narcissus, storax
Venus	Emerald green	Rose, myrtle, fennel, vervain, maidenhair	Copper	Emerald, turquoise	Ambergris, sandalwood, musk, benzoin, pink rose, myrtle
Mars	Scarlet	Absinth, rue, lamb's tongue	Iron	Ruby	Benzoin, sulphur, tobacco
Jupiter	Blue	Narcissus, oak, poplar, agrimony	Tin	Amethyst, sapphire	Nutmeg, cinnamon, balm, cloves, aloe wood
Saturn	Indigo	Ash, yew, cypress, house leek	Lead	Onyx, sapphire	Civet, musk, alum

* From Conway, D., 'Magic: An Occult Primer', The Aquarian Press, 1988

Bibliography

Agrippa, H. C., *La Philosophie Occulte* (1651), trans. John French, London, 1987.

Al-Kindi, *The Medical Formulary*, trans. M. Levey, Wisconsin Press, 1966.

Atchley, E. G. C. F., *The History and Uses of Incense in Divine Worship*, Longman Green, 1909.

Beckett., S., *Herbs to Soothe your Nerves*, Thorsons, 1977.

Bellamy, D. and Pfister, A., *World Medicine*, Blackwell, 1992.

Beresford-Cooke, C., *Massage: for Healing and Relaxation*, Arlington, 1986.

Bianchini, F. and Corbetta, F., *Health Plants of the World – Atlas of Medicinal Plants*, Newsweek Books, New York, 1977.

Boulos, C. and Danin, A., *Medicinal Plants of North Africa*, Reference Publications, 1983.

British Herbal Pharmacopoeia, *British Herbal Medicine Association, 1983.*

Buchman, D. D., *Herbal Medicine*, Rider, London, 1984.

Cabanis, P. J. G., *Oeuvres Completes*, Paris, 1956.

Carrington, H., *Perfumes: Their Sensual Lure and Charm*, Haldeman-Julius Publications, 1947.

Castrén, P., *Ancient and Popular Healing*, Vammalan Kirjapaino Oy, Vammala, 1989.

Chetwynd, T., *A Dictionary of Symbols*, Paladin, 1982.

Chiej, R., *The Macdonald Encyclopedia of Medicinal Plants*, Arnoldo Montadori Editore, Milan, 1984.

Cobb, N. and Loewe, E., *Sphinx 3, A Journal for Archetypal Psychology and the Arts*, Claughton Press, 1990.

Cohen, J. M., 'On Smells by Montaigne' in *Essays*, Penguin, 1958.

Comito, T., *The Idea of the Garden in the Renaissance*, Harvester Press, 1979.

Conway, D., *The Magic of Herbs*, Mayflower, 1973.

Coon, N., *The Dictionary of Useful Plants*, Rodale, Emmaus, 1974.

Cribb, A. B. and J. W., *Useful Wild Plants in Australia*, Fontana/Collins, 1982.

Culpeper, N., *Culpeper's Complete Herbal*, W. Foulsham & Co. Ltd.

Cunningham, S., *Magical Herbalism*, Llewellyn, 1956.

—, *Magical Aromatherapy*, Llewellyn, 1989.

Dastur, J. F., *Useful Plants of India and Pakistan*, D. B. Taraporevala, Sons & Co. Ltd., 1985.

Davis, J., *A Garden of Miracles*, Fredrick Muller, 1985.

Davis, P., *Aromatherapy: An A–Z*, C. W. Daniel, 1988.

—, *Subtle Aromatherapy*, C. W. Daniel, 1991.

Dawson, W. R., *Magician and Leech*, Methuen and Co., 1929.

Day, I., *Perfumery with Herbs*, Darton, Longman and Todd, 1979.

De Baïracli, Levy, J., *The Illustrated Herbal Handbook*, Faber & Faber, 1982.

De Rola, S. K., *Alchemy, The Secret Art*, Thames & Hudson, 1973.

Dobbs, B. J. T., *The Foundations of Newton's Alchemy*, Cambridge University Press, 1975.

Dodd, G. H. and Van Toller, S., *Perfumery: The Psychology and Biology of Fragrance I*, Chapman and Hall, 1990.

—, *Fragrance: The Psychology and Biology of Perfume II*, Elsevier Science Publications Ltd., 1992.

Douglas, J. S., *Making your own Cosmetics*, Pelham Books, 1979.

Fabricius, J., *Alchemy*, The Aquarian Press, 1976.

Fischer-Rizzi, S., *Complete Aromatherapy Handbook*, Sterling, 1990.

Franchomme, P., *Phytoguide*, no. 1., International Phytomedical Foundation.

Furia, T. E. and Bellanca, N., *Fenaroli's Handbook of Flavour Ingredients*, 2nd ed., Vol. 1., CRC Press, Cleveland, Ohio, 1975.

Gattefossé, R. M., *Gattefossé's Aromatherapy* 1937, reprinted C. W. Daniel, 1993.

Gerard, J., *The Herball or Generall Historie of Plants*, Thomas Johnson, London, 1633.

Ghalioungui, P., *Magic and Medical Science in Ancient Egypt*, Hodder & Stoughton, 1963.

Goodwin, G., *Scents and Aromatics*, The Gelofer Press, London, 1979.

Gordon, B. L., *The Romance of Medicine: The Story of the Evolution of Medicine from Occult Practices and Primitive Times*, F. A. Davis Co., Philadelphia, 1945.

Gordon, L., *A Country Herbal*, Webb & Bower, 1980.

Green, M. J., *The Gods of Roman Britain*, Shire Publications Ltd., 1983.

Grieve, M., *A Modern Herbal*, Penguin Books, Middlesex, 1982.

Griggs, B., *The Home Herbal*, Pan Books, London, 1983.

Grimm Brothers, *The Complete Grimm's Fairytales*, Routledge and Kegan Paul, 1975.

Groom, N., *Frankincense and Myrrh*, Longman, 1981.

—, *The Perfume Handbook*, Chapman and Hall, 1992.

Guenther, E., *The Essential Oils*, Van Nostrand, New York, 1948.

Gwilt, J., *Biblical Ills and Remedies*, The Society of Apothecaries of London, 1985.

Hall, D., *The Book of Herbs*, Angus and Robertson Publishers, 1972.

Haupt, P., 'Manna, Nectar and Ambrosia' in The American Philosophical Society *Proceedings*, Vol. LXI, No. 3, 1922.

Heriteau, J., *Potpourris and other Fragrant Delights*, Penguin, 1975.

Hilton-Simpson, M. W., *Some Arab and Shawia Remedies*, The Royal Anthropological Institute, 1913.

Hoffmann, D., *The Holistic Herbal*, Findhorn Press, 1983.

Howard, G., *The Principles and Practice of Perfumery and Cosmetics*, Stanley Thornes Ltd., 1987.

Jellinek, P., *The Practice of Modern Perfumery*, Leonard Hill, 1959.

Jessee, J. E., *Perfume Album*, Robert E., Krieger, 1974.

Jung, C. G., *The Collected Works*, trans R. R. C. Hull, Routledge and Kegan Paul.

Kemp, P., *Healing Rituals*, Faber and Faber, 1935.

Kenton, L., *Stress and Relaxation*, Windward, 1986.

Kenton, W., *Astrology: The Celestial Mirror*, Avon Books, 1974.

Khan, I., *The Development of Spiritual Healing*, Sufi Publishing Co., 1974.

King, J. R., *Have the Scents to Relax*, World Medicine, 1983.

Krochmal, A. and C., *A Guide to the Medicinal Plants of the United States*, Quadrangle, The New York Times Book Co., 1973.

Lake, M., *Scents and Sensuality*, Murray, 1989.

Larcher, H., *Le sang, peut-il vaincre la mort?*, Paris Gallimard, 1957.

Lassak, E. V. and McCarthy, T., *Australian Medicinal Plants*, Methuen, Australia, 1983.

Lautie, R, and Passebecq, A., *Aromatherapy: The Use of Plant Essences in Healing*, Thorsons, 1982.

Lavabre, M., *Aromatherapy Workbook*, Healing Arts Press, Vermont, 1990.

Lawless, J., *The Encyclopaedia of Essential Oils*, Element Books, 1992.

—, *Home Aromatherapy*, Kyle Cathie Ltd., 1993.

Lawrence, B. M., *Essential Oils*, Allured Publishing Co., Wheaton, 1978.

Le Guérer, A., *Scent: The Mysterious Power of Smell*, Chatto & Windus, 1993.

Le Strange, R., *A History of Herbal Plants*, Angus and Robertson, 1977.

Leung, A. Y., *Encyclopedia of Common Natural Ingredients*, John Wiley, New York, 1980.

Lewis, R. and Lowe, P., *Individual Excellence*, Kogan Page, 1992.

Lovell, R., *A Compleat Herball*, 2nd ed., London, 1665.

Manniche, L., *An Ancient Egyptian Herbal*, British Museum Publications, 1989.

Maury, M., *Marguerite Maury's Guide to Aromatherapy*, C. W. Daniel, 1989.

Maybe, R., *The Complete New Herbal*, Elm Tree Books, 1988.

McKenzie, D., *Aromatics and the Soul*, Heinemann, 1923.

Mendels, K. D., *Perfumes and Cosmetics in the Ancient World*, The Israel Museum, Jerusalem, 1989.

Metcalfe, J., *Herbs and Aromatherapy*, Webb & Bower, 1989.

Meunier, C., *Lavandes et Lavandins*, Charly-Yves Chaudoreille, Edisud, 1985.

Miller, R. A. and I., *The Magical and Ritual Use of Perfumes*, Destiny Books, USA, 1990.

Mills, S. Y., *The A–Z of Modern Herbalism*, Thorsons, 1989.

Morris, E. T., *Fragrance: The Story of Perfume from Cleopatra to Chanel*, Charles Scribner's Sons, New York.

Moyers, B., *Healing and the Mind*, Thorsons, 1993.

Muller, P. M. and Lamparsky, D., *Perfumes, Art, Science, Technology*, Elsevier Applied Science, 1991.

Myerhoff, B., *American Folk Medicine*, University of California Press, 1976.

Naves, Y. R. and Mazuyer, G., *Natural Perfume Materials*, Reinhold Publishing, New York, 1947.

Nefzawi, Shaykh, *The Perfumed Garden*, trans. Sir Richard Burton, Neville Spearman Ltd., 1963.

Nielsen, K., *Incense in Ancient Israel*, E. J. Brill, 1986.

Norbu, N., *On Birth and Life: A Treatise on Tibetan Medicine*, Shang-shung Edizioni, 1983.

Omont, A., 'Les molecules aromatiques de milieu interstellaire' in *Aux Frontières de la Science*, La Recherche, 1989.

Page, M., *The Observer's Book of Herbs*, Frederick Warne, 1980.

Parvati, J., *Hygieia, A Woman's Herbal*, Wildwood House, London, 1979.

Phillips, R., *Wild Flowers of Britain*, Pan Books, 1977.

Pliny, C., *The History of Nature*, trans. H. Rackham, London, 1938.

Pomet, P., *A Compleat History of Druggs*, Lemery & Tournefort, 1712.

Poucher, W. A., *Perfumes, Cosmetics and Soaps*, Vol. II, Chapman and Hall, 1932.

Powell, N., *Alchemy: The Ancient Science*, Aldus Books, 1976.

Poynter and Keele, *A Short History of Medicine*, Mills & Boon, 1961.

Price, S., *Practical Aromatherapy*, Thorsons, 1983.

Rapgay, L., *Tibetan Therapeutic Massage*, published by the author, India, 1985.

Ranson, F., *British Herbs*, Penguin, 1949.

Rather, L. J., *Mind and Body in 18th Century Medicine*, Wellcome Historical Medical Library, 1965.

Robbins, T., *Jitterbug Perfume*, Bantham, 1984.

Roudnitska, E., *The Art of Perfumery*, Cabris, France.

Ryman, D., *The Aromatherapy Handbook*, Century, 1984.

—, *Aromatherapy*, Piatkus, 1991.

Shelmerdine, C. W., *The Perfume Industry of Mycenaean Pylos*, P. A. Forlag, 1985.

Sigismund, R., *Die Aromata*, C. F. Winterische Verlagshandlung, Leipzig, 1884.

Stead, C., *The Power of Holistic Aromatherapy*, Javelin Books, 1986.

Stobart, T., *Herbs, Spices and Flavourings*, Penguin, 1979.

Stoddart, D. M., *The Scented Ape*, Cambridge University Press, 1990.

Süskind, P., *Perfume: The Story of a Murderer*, Hamish Hamilton, London, 1986.

Sutcliffe, J., The Complete Book of Relaxation Techniques, Headline, 1991.

Theophrastus, *Enquiry into Plants*, Leyden, 1613.

Thompson, C. J. S., *The Mystery and Lure of Perfume*, John Lane, 1927.

Thomson, W. A. R., *Healing Plants – A Modern Herbal*, Macmillan, 1978.

Tisserand, M., *Aromatherapy for Women*, Thorsons, 1985.

—, *Aromatherapy for Lovers*, Thorsons, 1993.

Tisserand, R., *The Essential Oil Safety Data Manual*, The Association of Tisserand Aromatherapists, 1985.

—, *The Art of Aromatherapy*, C. W. Daniel, 1985.

Valnet, J., *The Practice of Aromatherapy*, English translation, C .W. Daniel, 1982.

Von Staden, *Herophilus: The Art of Medicine in Early Alexandria*, Cambridge University Press, 1989.

Waite, A. E., *The Hermetic and Alchemical Writings of Paracelsus*, Vols I and II, T. Elliott & Co., Berkeley, 1976.

Ware, J. R., trans., *Alchemy, Medicine and Religion in the China of AD 320, The*, M.I.T. Press, 1966.

Weiss, R. F., *Herbal Medicine*, Arcanum, 1988.

Whitebread, C., *The Magic, Psychic, Ancient Egyptian, Greek and Roman Medical Collections*, U.S. National Museum, 1924.

Whitmont, E. C., *Psyche and Substance*, North Atlantic Books, 1980.

—, *The Return of the Goddess*, Routledge and Kegan Paul, 1983.

Wildwood, C., *Creative Aromatherapy*, Thorsons, 1993.

Williams, D., *Lecture Notes on Essential Oils*, Eve Taylor Ltd., 1989.

Worwood, V. A., *The Fragrant Pharmacy*, Macmillan, 1990.

—, *Aromatics*, reprinted Bantam Books, 1993.

Wright, R., *The Science of Smell*, Allen and Unwin, 1964.

Wren, R. C., *Potters New Cyclopaedia of Botanical Drugs and Preparations*, C. W. Daniel, 1988.

Younger, D., *Household Gods*, E. W. Allen, London, 1898.

INDEX